GOUT DIET

COOKBOOK FOR SENIORS

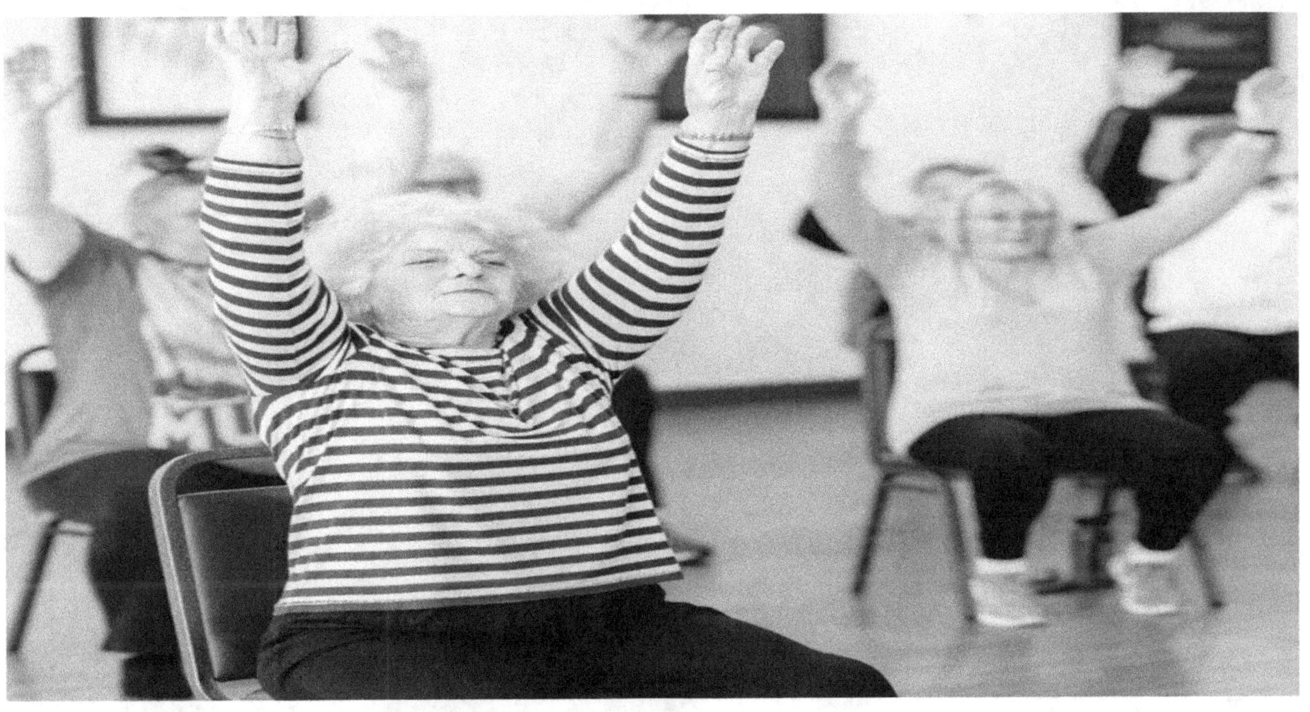

Low-Purine Diet: Delicious Recipes and a Guide to Anti-Inflammatory Natural Foods

Luna Hartfield

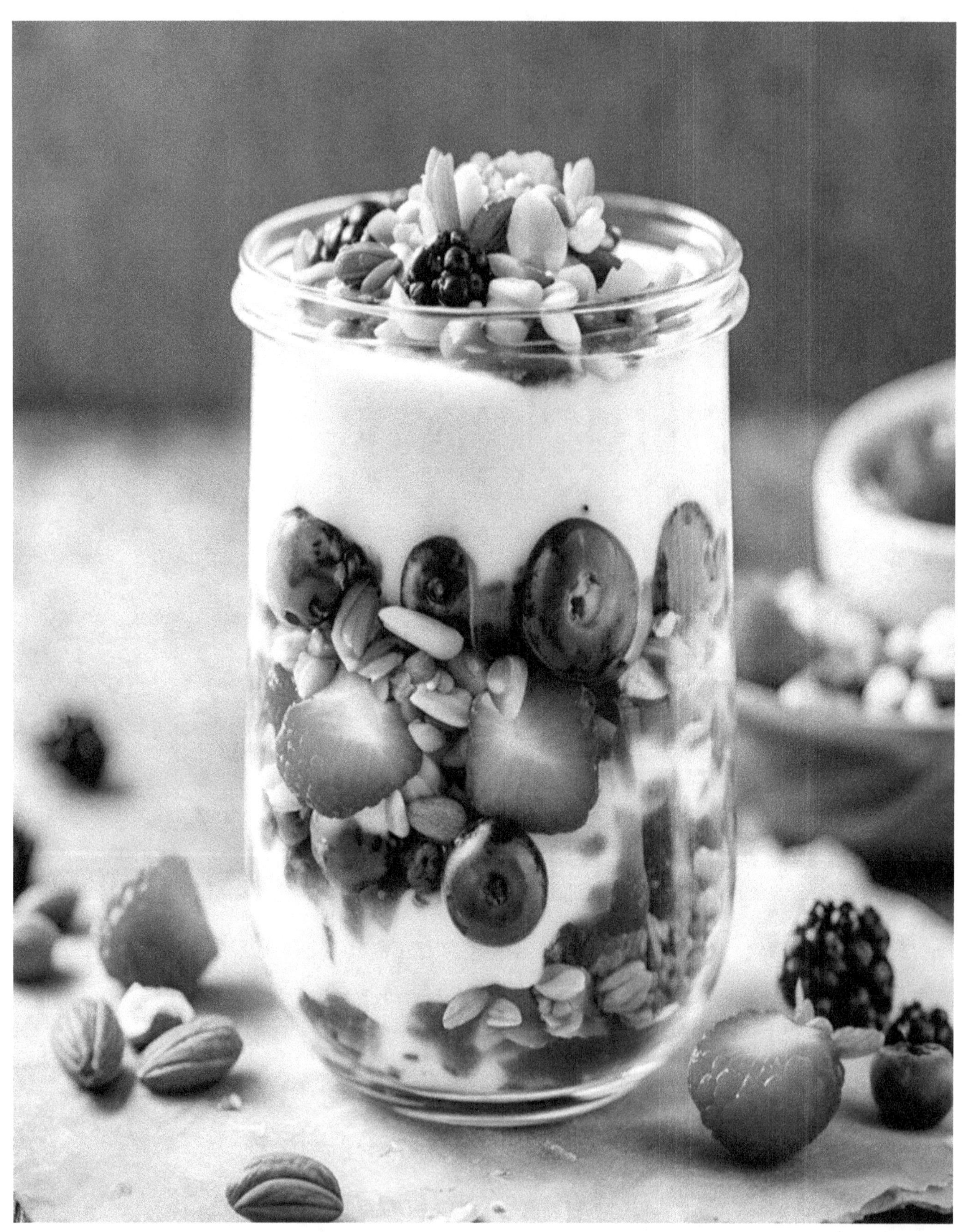

Copyright © *Luna Hartfield*, 2024.

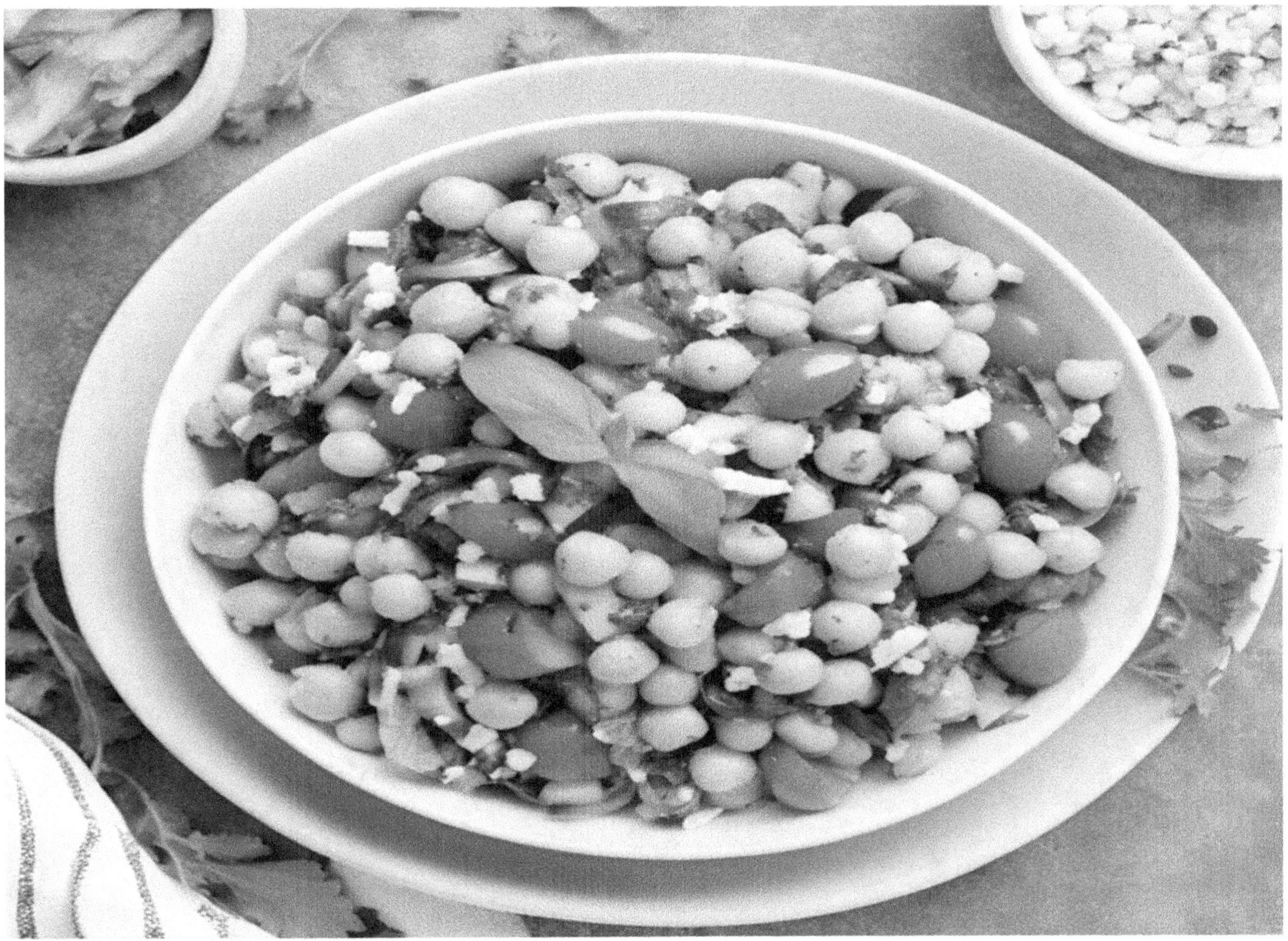

TABLE OF CONTENTS

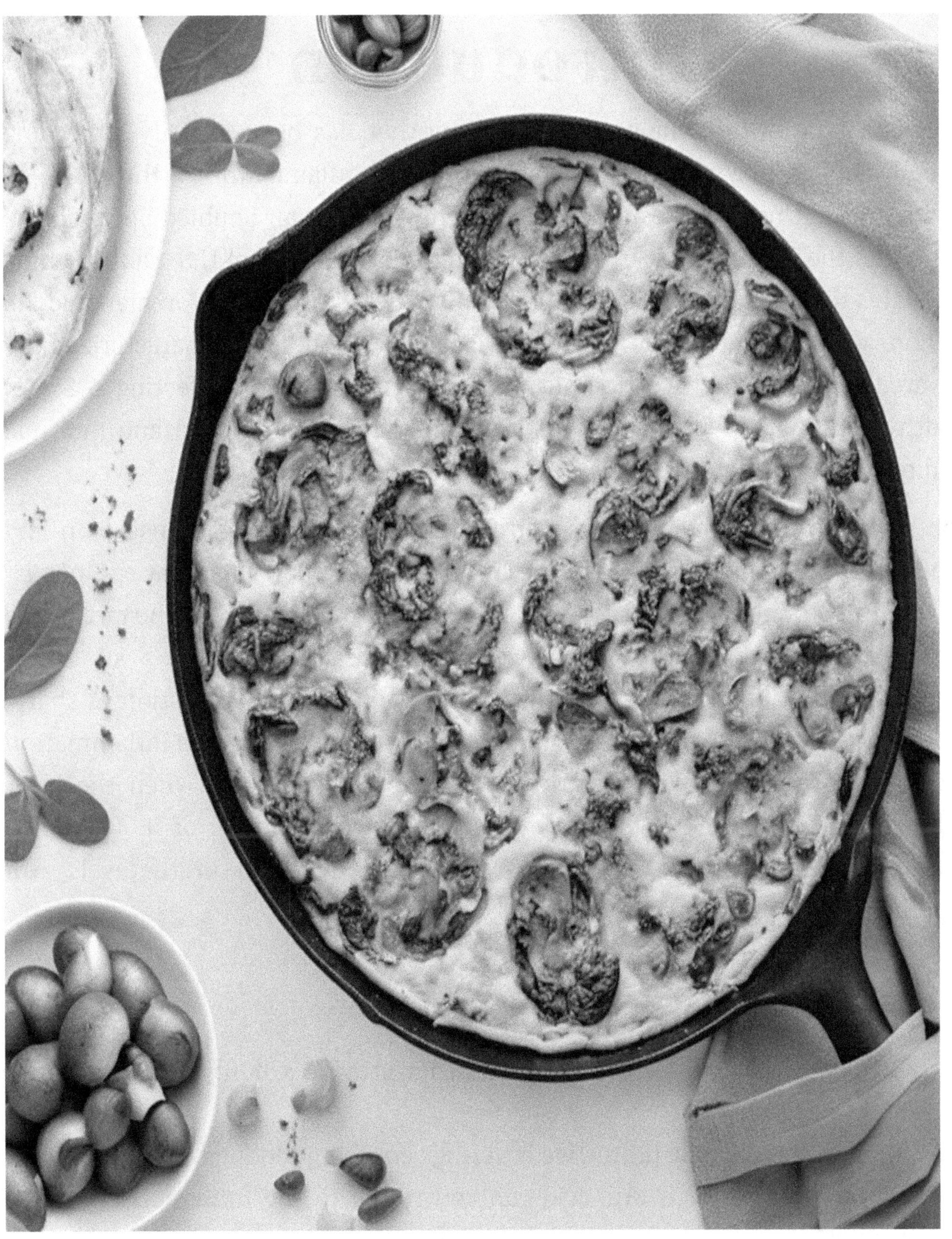

Introduction

Gout is a type of inflammatory arthropathy that has been steadily increasing globally and is now the most common type of inflammatory arthropathy in adults. In the United States, its prevalence has more than doubled between the 1960s and the 1990s, and it is now estimated to affect 3.9% of U.S. adults, which translates to approximately 8.3 million adults, including 6.1 million men and 2.2 million women. Furthermore, hyperuricemia, a condition characterized by elevated levels of uric acid in the blood, is also prevalent, affecting 6-8% of healthy adults and 1 in 3 adults with uncontrolled hypertension and multiple cardiovascular risk factors.

Gout is a form of inflammatory arthritis known for causing intense pain and swelling in the joints, typically in the form of sudden flare-ups that can persist for one to two weeks before subsiding. These painful episodes often start in the big toe or a lower extremity. The condition arises when there's an excess accumulation of urate in the body over time, leading to the formation of sharp, needle-like crystals in and around the affected joint, which causes inflammation and joint pain associated with arthritis. This build-up occurs when the body either produces too much urate or doesn't eliminate enough of it. It's worth noting, though, that not everyone with elevated serum urate levels will experience gout.

Gout can impact various body parts, including:

- Joints.
- Bursae, which are the cushiony sacs that provide a buffer between bones and soft tissues.
- Tendon sheaths, the protective coverings encasing tendons.
- Kidneys, where high uric acid can contribute to the formation of kidney stones.

Who's likely to get gout?

It's a condition that affects many, with a higher prevalence in men than women. Gout typically shows up in middle age for men, while women are generally at lower risk until after menopause, meaning they tend to get it later in life. It's less common in younger individuals, but when it does occur, it can be particularly severe.

How long does a gout attack last?

Well, these attacks often stick around for a week or two. Some flares might linger a bit longer or hit with more intensity. In the periods between these attacks, you might not feel any symptoms at all.

How is gout diagnosed?

To determine if someone has gout, a medical professional will conduct a physical assessment, inquire about the individual's symptoms, and inspect the joints that are causing discomfort. It's important to share with your doctor when you first noticed signs such as pain and swelling, and how frequently these symptoms have been occurring.

What tests will be done to diagnose gout?

To confirm a diagnosis of gout, your doctor may use several imaging techniques to get a clearer view of the affected joints and to check for any damage caused by the condition. These imaging tests can include:

- X-rays to look at the bone structure.
- Ultrasound to detect urate crystals.
- MRI to provide detailed images of the soft tissues.
- Dual-energy CT scans to identify urate crystals with precision.

Additionally, other diagnostic tests for gout are:

- Blood tests to measure the levels of uric acid.

- Joint fluid analysis, where fluid is drawn from the joint with a needle for examination.

Management and Treatment

When it comes to treatment, gout is typically managed with a two-pronged approach: addressing the immediate symptoms during a flare-up and making dietary adjustments to reduce intake of foods and beverages high in purines.

Gout medication

Medications are often prescribed to alleviate gout symptoms, such as:

- **NSAIDs:** These over-the-counter drugs, like ibuprofen and naproxen, can help ease pain and reduce inflammation. However, if you have conditions like kidney disease or stomach ulcers, consult your doctor before taking NSAIDs.
- **Colchicine:** This prescription drug can significantly decrease inflammation and pain when taken at the onset of a gout attack, ideally within the first 24 hours.
- **Corticosteroids:** Available as oral medications or injections, corticosteroids can be administered directly into the joint or given intramuscularly to combat inflammation. Your doctor will decide the best form of administration based on your specific needs.

Gout is caused by the accumulation of urate crystals in the joints, which triggers inflammation and intense pain. This accumulation occurs due to high levels of uric acid in the blood. Various factors can contribute to increased uric acid levels and the development of gout:

1. **Dietary Factors**:

   - **High-Purine Foods**: Consuming foods rich in purines, such as red meat, organ meats (liver, kidneys), and certain types of seafood (anchovies, sardines, mussels, scallops, trout, and tuna) can raise uric acid levels.

   - **Sugary Beverages**: Drinks sweetened with fructose, such as soda and fruit juices, can increase uric acid production.

   - **Alcohol**: Beer and distilled liquors are known to elevate uric acid levels.

2. **Medical Conditions**:

   - **Obesity**: Excess body weight is associated with higher uric acid production and decreased ability to excrete it.

   - **Hypertension**: High blood pressure can be linked to higher uric acid levels.

   - **Diabetes**: Insulin resistance associated with diabetes can lead to increased uric acid.

   - **Metabolic Syndrome**: A cluster of conditions, including increased blood pressure, high blood sugar, excess body fat around the waist, and abnormal cholesterol levels, can increase the risk of gout.

   - **Kidney Diseases**: Reduced kidney function can lead to inefficient uric acid excretion.

3. **Genetics**:

- **Family History**: A family history of gout can increase the likelihood of developing the condition, suggesting a genetic predisposition.

4. **Medications**:

- **Diuretics (Water Pills)**: Used to treat hypertension and other conditions, diuretics can increase uric acid levels.

- **Low-Dose Aspirin**: Regular use of low-dose aspirin can affect uric acid excretion.

- **Immunosuppressants**: Drugs such as cyclosporine can raise uric acid levels.

5. **Other Factors**:

- **Age and Sex**: Gout is more common in men than in women, primarily because women tend to have lower uric acid levels. However, women's uric acid levels approach those of men after menopause. Gout typically occurs in men between the ages of 30 and 50, while it tends to develop later in women.

- **Recent Surgery or Trauma**: Physical stress can sometimes trigger a gout attack.

- **Dehydration**: Not drinking enough fluids can increase uric acid concentration in the blood.

Gout symptoms typically appear suddenly and can cause significant discomfort. The main symptoms include:

1. **Severe Joint Pain**:

   - The pain often starts suddenly, typically at night, and is most severe within the first 4 to 12 hours.

   - It commonly affects the large joint of the big toe, but it can also occur in other joints, such as the ankles, knees, elbows, wrists, and fingers.

2. **Lingering Discomfort**:

   - After the most severe pain subsides, some joint discomfort may last from a few days to a few weeks.

   - Subsequent attacks are likely to last longer and affect more joints.

3. **Inflammation and Redness**:

   - The affected joint or joints become swollen, tender, and red.

   - The area around the joint may be warm to the touch.

4. **Limited Range of Motion**:

   - As gout progresses, it can limit the movement in the affected joints.

   - Joint stiffness and reduced flexibility can occur during and between attacks.

5. **Tophi Development**:

   - Over time, urate crystals can form lumps called tophi, which can develop under the skin around affected joints.

   - Tophi can also occur in other areas, such as the fingers, hands, feet, elbows, and Achilles tendons.

6. **Fever**:

- In some cases, individuals with a severe gout attack may develop a mild fever.

Stages of Gout

1. **Asymptomatic Hyperuricemia**:

- High levels of uric acid are present in the blood, but no symptoms are experienced.
- This stage can last for many years before progressing to acute gout.

2. **Acute Gout**:

- This stage is characterized by sudden and severe attacks of pain and inflammation in one or more joints.
- The pain typically occurs at night and is most intense in the first 12-24 hours.

3. **Intercritical Gout**:

- This stage refers to the periods between acute gout attacks, during which there are no symptoms.
- Without treatment, these symptom-free periods become shorter, and attacks may become more frequent and severe.

4. **Chronic Tophaceous Gout**:

- This is the most severe form of gout, occurring after many years of recurrent acute attacks.
- It is characterized by persistent joint pain, damage to the joints and surrounding tissues, and the presence of tophi.
- Chronic gout can lead to deformities and disability if not properly managed.

Alcoholic Beverages:

- Beer and grain liquors (such as vodka and whiskey)

Meats:

- Red meat (beef, lamb, pork)
- Organ meats (liver, kidneys, and glandular meats like the thymus or pancreas, often referred to as sweetbreads)

Seafood:

- Shellfish (shrimp, lobster, mussels)
- Fish (anchovies, sardines, Coldwater fish)

High-Fructose Foods and Beverages:

- Soda and some juices
- Cereals
- Ice cream
- Candy
- Fast food

Other Foods:

- Yeast extract
- Sugary foods and beverages
- White bread
- Honey

Low-Fat and Non-Dairy Fat Products:

- Yogurt and skim milk

Fruits and Vegetables:

- Fresh fruits and vegetables

- Citrus fruits

- Cherries or 100% cherry juice

- Vegetables like spinach and asparagus (studies show they don't increase gout risk)

Protein Sources:

- Nuts, peanut butter, and grains

- Eggs (in moderation)

- Meats like fish, chicken, and red meat in moderation (about 4 to 6 ounces per day)

- Tofu

- Beans and lentils

Carbohydrates:

- Potatoes, rice, bread, and pasta

- Whole grains

Fats and Oils:

- Plant-based oils

- Fat and oil

- Avocados

Beverages:

- Coffee

Dairy Products:

- Various dairy products

The Role of Diet in Managing Gout

Diet plays a crucial role in managing gout, as certain foods can either trigger or help prevent gout flare-ups. Here's how diet impacts gout management:

1. **Reducing Uric Acid Levels**:

   - **Low-Purine Diet**: Purines are substances found in certain foods that the body breaks down into uric acid. A diet low in purines can help reduce uric acid levels in the blood.

   - **Foods to Avoid**: High-purine foods, such as red meat, organ meats, and certain types of seafood (like anchovies, sardines, and mackerel), should be limited or avoided.

   - **Alcohol and Sugary Beverages**: Limiting or avoiding alcohol (especially beer and spirits) and sugary beverages, such as sodas and fruit juices, can help lower uric acid levels.

2. **Encouraging Foods that Help Manage Gout**:

   - **Low-Purine Foods**: Emphasizing low-purine foods, such as fruits, vegetables, whole grains, and low-fat dairy products, can help manage gout.

   - **Cherries**: Some studies suggest that cherries and cherry juice may help reduce the frequency of gout attacks.

   - **Coffee**: Moderate coffee consumption may be associated with a lower risk of gout.

3. **Promoting Anti-Inflammatory Foods**:

- **Omega-3 Fatty Acids**: Foods rich in omega-3 fatty acids, such as flaxseeds, chia seeds, and fatty fish (like salmon and mackerel), have anti-inflammatory properties.

- **Fruits and Vegetables**: Many fruits and vegetables are rich in antioxidants and can help reduce inflammation. Berries, cherries, and citrus fruits are particularly beneficial.

- **Herbs and Spices**: Turmeric and ginger have potent anti-inflammatory effects and can be included in a gout-friendly diet.

4. **Maintaining a Healthy Weight**:

- **Weight Management**: Obesity is a risk factor for gout. A balanced diet that helps achieve and maintain a healthy weight can reduce the frequency and severity of gout attacks.

- **Caloric Balance**: Focus on a diet that balances caloric intake with energy expenditure to prevent weight gain.

5. **Staying Hydrated**:

- **Adequate Hydration**: Drinking plenty of water helps the kidneys flush out uric acid more efficiently. Aim for at least 8-12 cups of water per day.

- **Avoiding Dehydration**: Dehydration can increase uric acid concentration in the blood, so it's important to stay well-hydrated.

6. **Meal Planning and Portion Control**:

- **Regular Meals**: Eating regular, balanced meals helps maintain stable blood sugar levels and prevents overeating.

- **Portion Sizes**: Controlling portion sizes can help manage weight and reduce the risk of gout attacks.

The Gout diet

Gout happens when uric acid gets too cozy in your bloodstream, turning into annoying crystals that crash at your joint's place, causing pain and swelling. To kick out these uninvited guests, you can switch to a diet that's low on purines, which is like not giving them any snacks to munch on. Fewer purines mean fewer crystals, and that means fewer gout flare-ups.

What is a low purine diet?

Think of purines as the party fuel for uric acid. They're in a bunch of foods and drinks, and when they break down, they leave uric acid behind. Go easy on the purines, and your body says "thanks" by lowering the uric acid levels. Plus, some foods are like bouncers, helping to show uric acid to the door.

Who can benefit from a low-purine diet?

If your body's uric acid is like a crowd-surfing fan at a concert (a.k.a. hyperuricemia), a low-purine diet could be your backstage pass to preventing gout or keeping it from getting worse. It's also a good move for dodging other hyperuricemia hits, like kidney stones.

Risks / Benefits

What are the advantages of a low-purine diet?

- **Less uric acid:** If you're prone to hyperuricemia, tweaking your diet could keep things like gout and kidney stones from crashing your party. If you've already got gout, it could stop more crystals from forming.
- **Drop some pounds:** Kicking high-purine grub to the curb often means saying goodbye to stuff like red meat and sugary treats, which can also lead to weight loss. Since being overweight is like a VIP pass for gout, slimming down can help ease your joints and cut your gout risk.
- **Ease up on meds:** While diet isn't a stand-in for meds, it might help you use less of them.

- **It's limiting:** A low-purine life means parting ways with some beloved treats, like sugary snacks and alcohol. Sticking to it can be tough, especially since it's more of a sidekick to medication rather than the hero.
- **It limits omega-3 sources:** Seafood's got those omega-3s that chill out inflammation, but it's also got purines. The good news is you can still get your omega-3 fix with fish oil supplements.
- **It's not a cure:** Diet alone won't drop your uric acid levels like meds can. The best play is to team them up. Some folks question if the diet's worth it compared to meds, but often, meds need a diet friend to tackle gout.

Gout home remedies

Sure thing! Some folks find that these goodies might help keep uric acid on the down low and fend off gout attacks:

- Sour cherries
- A dash of magnesium
- Ginger
- A splash of diluted apple cider vinegar
- Crunchy celery
- A cup of nettle tea
- Dandelion greens
- Milk thistle seeds

Remember, these are just friendly neighborhood advice and not a substitute for professional medical guidance. If gouts got you down, have a chat with your doc to figure out the best game plan for you.

Breakfast Recipes

Almond Butter and Banana Whole Wheat Toast

Prep Time: 5 minutes | **Cook Time**: 0 minutes | **Total Time**: 5 minutes | **Per Serving**: 2 servings

Ingredients:

- 2 slices whole wheat bread, toasted
- 2 tablespoons almond butter
- 1 banana, sliced
- 1 teaspoon honey (optional)
- A pinch of cinnamon (optional)

Instructions:

1. Spread 1 tablespoon of almond butter on each slice of toasted whole wheat bread.
2. Arrange the banana slices on top of the almond butter.
3. Drizzle with honey and sprinkle with cinnamon if desired.
4. Serve immediately.

Nutritional Value: Calories: 250 | Phosphorus: 3g | Sodium: 5g | Protein: 6g | Carbohydrates: 35g | Fats: 10g | Potassium: 4g | Iron: 5g

Greek Yogurt Parfait with Berries and Nuts

Prep Time: 10 minutes | **Cook Time**: 0 minutes | **Total Time**: 10 minutes | **Per Serving**: 2 servings

Ingredients:

- 2 cups Greek yogurt
- 1 cup mixed berries (blueberries, strawberries, raspberries)
- 1/4 cup granola
- 2 tablespoons chopped nuts (almonds, walnuts)
- 1 tablespoon honey (optional)

Instructions:

1. In a glass or bowl, layer 1/2 cup of Greek yogurt.
2. Add a layer of mixed berries, followed by a tablespoon of granola and nuts.
3. Repeat the layers and top with honey if desired.
4. Serve immediately.

Nutritional Value: Calories: 280 | Phosphorus: 4g | Sodium: 6g | Protein: 12g | Carbohydrates: 30g | Fats: 10g | Potassium: 5g | Iron: 5g

Spinach and Mushroom Frittata

Prep Time: 10 minutes | **Cook Time**: 20 minutes | **Total Time**: 30 minutes | **Per Serving**: 4 servings

Ingredients:

- 6 large eggs
- 1/4 cup milk
- 1 cup fresh spinach, chopped
- 1 cup mushrooms, sliced
- 1/2 cup onion, diced
- 1/2 cup shredded cheese (optional)
- 1 tablespoon olive oil
- Salt and pepper, to taste

Instructions:

1. Preheat oven to 375°F (190°C).
2. In a bowl, whisk together eggs, milk, salt, and pepper.
3. In an oven-safe skillet, heat olive oil over medium heat. Add onions and mushrooms, and sauté until soft.
4. Add spinach and cook until wilted.
5. Pour the egg mixture over the vegetables and cook for a few minutes until the edges start to set.
6. Sprinkle cheese on top if using.
7. Transfer the skillet to the oven and bake for 10-12 minutes, or until the frittata is fully set.
8. Remove from the oven, let cool slightly, slice, and serve.

Nutritional Value: Calories: 200 | Phosphorus: 6g | Sodium: 7g | Protein: 14g | Carbohydrates: 8g | Fats: 15g | Potassium: 4g | Iron: 6g

Steel-Cut Oats with Cinnamon and Apples

Prep Time: 5 minutes | **Cook Time**: 30 minutes | **Total Time**: 35 minutes | **Per Serving**: 4 servings

Ingredients:

- 1 cup steel-cut oats
- 4 cups water
- 1 apple, diced
- 1 teaspoon ground cinnamon
- 1/4 teaspoon salt
- 1 tablespoon honey (optional)
- 1/4 cup chopped walnuts (optional)

Instructions:

1. In a medium saucepan, bring water to a boil. Add salt and steel-cut oats.
2. Reduce heat and simmer for about 25-30 minutes, stirring occasionally.
3. During the last 5 minutes of cooking, add diced apple and cinnamon.
4. Remove from heat, stir in honey and walnuts if desired.
5. Serve hot.

Nutritional Value: Calories: 220 | Phosphorus: 4g | Sodium: 5g | Protein: 6g | Carbohydrates: 40g | Fats: 6g | Potassium: 4g | Iron: 5g

Sweet Potato Hash with Bell Peppers

Prep Time: 10 minutes | **Cook Time**: 20 minutes | **Total Time**: 30 minutes | **Per Serving**: 4 servings

Ingredients:

- 2 medium sweet potatoes, peeled and diced
- 1 red bell pepper, diced
- 1 green bell pepper, diced
- 1 small onion, diced
- 2 tablespoons olive oil
- 1 teaspoon smoked paprika
- Salt and pepper, to taste
- 2 tablespoons fresh parsley, chopped (optional)

Instructions:

1. In a large skillet, heat olive oil over medium heat.
2. Add diced sweet potatoes and cook for about 10 minutes, stirring occasionally, until they begin to soften.
3. Add bell peppers and onion and cook for another 10 minutes until all vegetables are tender.
4. Stir in smoked paprika, salt, and pepper.
5. Garnish with fresh parsley if desired and serve immediately.

Nutritional Value: Calories: 180 | Phosphorus: 3g | Sodium: 4g | Protein: 2g | Carbohydrates: 30g | Fats: 7g | Potassium: 5g | Iron: 3g

Cherry Almond Overnight Oats

Prep Time: 10 minutes | **Cook Time**: 0 minutes | **Total Time**: 10 minutes (plus overnight chilling) | **Per Serving**: 2 servings

Ingredients:

- 1 cup rolled oats
- 1 cup almond milk
- 1/2 cup Greek yogurt
- 1/2 cup cherries, pitted and chopped
- 2 tablespoons chia seeds
- 1 tablespoon honey
- 1/4 teaspoon almond extract
- 2 tablespoons sliced almonds

Instructions:

1. In a bowl, mix oats, almond milk, Greek yogurt, cherries, chia seeds, honey, and almond extract.
2. Divide mixture into two jars or containers.
3. Refrigerate overnight.
4. In the morning, top with sliced almonds before serving.

Nutritional Value: Calories: 300 | Phosphorus: 4g | Sodium: 5g | Protein: 8g | Carbohydrates: 45g | Fats: 10g | Potassium: 4g | Iron: 3g

Avocado Toast with Smoked Salmon

Prep Time: 10 minutes | **Cook Time**: 0 minutes | **Total Time**: 10 minutes | **Per Serving**: 2 servings

Ingredients:

- 2 slices whole grain bread, toasted
- 1 ripe avocado, mashed
- 2 ounces smoked salmon
- 1/2 lemon, juiced
- Salt and pepper, to taste
- 1 tablespoon capers (optional)
- Fresh dill, for garnish (optional)

Instructions:

1. Spread mashed avocado evenly on toasted bread slices.
2. Drizzle with lemon juice and season with salt and pepper.
3. Top with smoked salmon and capers if using.
4. Garnish with fresh dill if desired.
5. Serve immediately.

Nutritional Value: Calories: 250 | Phosphorus: 3g | Sodium: 6g | Protein: 10g | Carbohydrates: 20g | Fats: 15g | Potassium: 5g | Iron: 3g

Egg White and Vegetable Wrap

Prep Time: 10 minutes | **Cook Time**: 10 minutes | **Total Time**: 20 minutes | **Per Serving**: 2 servings

Ingredients:

- 4 large egg whites

- 1/2 cup bell pepper, diced

- 1/2 cup spinach, chopped

- 1/4 cup onion, diced

- 1 tablespoon olive oil

- 2 whole wheat tortillas

- Salt and pepper, to taste

- 1/4 cup shredded cheese (optional)

Instructions:

1. In a skillet, heat olive oil over medium heat. Add onion and bell pepper, and sauté until tender.

2. Add spinach and cook until wilted.

3. Pour in egg whites and cook, stirring gently, until fully cooked. Season with salt and pepper.

4. Divide egg mixture between tortillas. Sprinkle with cheese if desired.

5. Roll up the tortillas and serve immediately.

Nutritional Value: Calories: 200 | Phosphorus: 4g | Sodium: 6g | Protein: 12g | Carbohydrates: 20g | Fats: 8g | Potassium: 3g | Iron: 4g

Quinoa Breakfast Bowl with Mango

Prep Time: 10 minutes | **Cook Time**: 15 minutes | **Total Time**: 25 minutes | **Per Serving**: 2 servings

Ingredients:

- 1 cup cooked quinoa
- 1/2 cup Greek yogurt
- 1 mango, peeled and diced
- 2 tablespoons chia seeds
- 1 tablespoon honey
- 1/4 teaspoon vanilla extract
- 1/4 cup shredded coconut

Instructions:

1. In a bowl, mix cooked quinoa, Greek yogurt, chia seeds, honey, and vanilla extract.
2. Divide the mixture into two bowls.
3. Top with diced mango and shredded coconut.
4. Serve immediately.

Nutritional Value: Calories: 320 | Phosphorus: 4g | Sodium: 5g | Protein: 10g | Carbohydrates: 50g | Fats: 10g | Potassium: 5g | Iron: 4g

Zucchini Bread Muffins

Prep Time: 15 minutes | **Cook Time**: 20 minutes | **Total Time**: 35 minutes | **Per Serving**: 12 muffins

Ingredients:

- 1 1/2 cups grated zucchini
- 1 1/2 cups whole wheat flour
- 1/2 cup rolled oats
- 1/2 cup brown sugar
- 1/4 cup olive oil
- 1/4 cup applesauce
- 2 large eggs
- 1 teaspoon vanilla extract
- 1 teaspoon baking powder
- 1/2 teaspoon baking soda
- 1/2 teaspoon ground cinnamon
- 1/4 teaspoon salt

Instructions:

1. Preheat oven to 350°F (175°C). Grease a muffin tin or line with paper liners.

2. In a large bowl, mix flour, oats, baking powder, baking soda, cinnamon, and salt.

3. In another bowl, beat eggs, then add brown sugar, olive oil, applesauce, and vanilla extract. Mix well.

4. Stir in grated zucchini.

5. Add the wet ingredients to the dry ingredients and mix until just combined.

6. Spoon the batter into the prepared muffin tin.

7. Bake for 18-20 minutes, or until a toothpick inserted into the center comes out clean.

8. Let muffins cool in the tin for 5 minutes, then transfer to a wire rack to cool completely.

Nutritional Value: Calories: 150 | Phosphorus: 3g | Sodium: 5g | Protein: 4g | Carbohydrates: 25g | Fats: 6g | Potassium: 3g | Iron: 3g

Vegetarians and Salads

Mediterranean Chickpea Salad

Prep Time: 15 minutes | **Cook Time**: 0 minutes | **Total Time**: 15 minutes | **Per Serving**: 4 servings

Ingredients:

- 2 cans (15 ounces each) chickpeas, drained and rinsed
- 1 cup cherry tomatoes, halved
- 1/2 English cucumber, diced
- 1/2 red onion, thinly sliced
- 1/2 cup Kalamata olives, pitted
- 1/4 cup fresh parsley, chopped
- 1/4 cup fresh mint, chopped
- 2 tablespoons extra virgin olive oil
- 2 tablespoons lemon juice
- 1 clove garlic, minced
- Salt and pepper, to taste
- Crumbled feta cheese, for serving (optional)

Instructions:

1. In a large bowl, combine the chickpeas, cherry tomatoes, cucumber, red onion, olives, parsley, and mint.

2. In a small bowl, whisk together the olive oil, lemon juice, garlic, salt, and pepper.

3. Pour the dressing over the chickpea mixture and toss until well combined.

4. Taste and adjust seasoning if necessary.

5. Serve the salad immediately, topped with crumbled feta cheese if desired.

Nutritional Value: Calories: 290 | Phosphorus: 5g | Sodium: 10g | Protein: 10g | Carbohydrates: 25g | Fats: 8g | Potassium: 5g | Iron: 8g

---

Grilled Tofu with Pineapple Salsa

Prep Time: 20 minutes | **Cook Time**: 10 minutes | **Total Time**: 30 minutes | **Per Serving**: 4 servings

Ingredients:

- 1 block (14 ounces) firm tofu, pressed and sliced
- 1 tablespoon olive oil
- Salt and pepper, to taste
- 1 cup fresh pineapple, diced
- 1/2 red bell pepper, diced
- 1/4 red onion, finely chopped
- 1 jalapeño, seeded and minced
- 1/4 cup fresh cilantro, chopped
- 2 tablespoons lime juice

Instructions:

1. Preheat the grill to medium-high heat.
2. Brush tofu slices with olive oil and season with salt and pepper.
3. Grill the tofu for 3-4 minutes on each side, until grill marks appear.
4. While the tofu is grilling, prepare the pineapple salsa by combining pineapple, red bell pepper, red onion, jalapeño, cilantro, and lime juice in a bowl.

5. Serve the grilled tofu topped with pineapple salsa.

Nutritional Value: Calories: 200 | Phosphorus: 4g | Sodium: 5g | Protein: 10g | Carbohydrates: 15g | Fats: 10g | Potassium: 4g | Iron: 6g

---

Roasted Beet and Orange Salad

Prep Time: 10 minutes | **Cook Time**: 30 minutes | **Total Time**: 40 minutes | **Per Serving**: 4 servings

Ingredients:

- 4 medium beets, roasted and sliced
- 2 oranges, peeled and segmented
- 1/4 red onion, thinly sliced
- 1/4 cup walnuts, toasted
- 2 tablespoons balsamic vinegar
- 2 tablespoons extra virgin olive oil
- Salt and pepper, to taste
- 2 tablespoons fresh mint, chopped

Instructions:

1. Preheat the oven to 400°F (200°C). Wrap beets in foil and roast for 30-40 minutes, until tender. Allow to cool, then peel and slice.

2. In a large bowl, combine roasted beets, orange segments, and red onion.

3. In a small bowl, whisk together balsamic vinegar, olive oil, salt, and pepper.

4. Pour dressing over the salad and toss gently.

5. Sprinkle with toasted walnuts and fresh mint before serving.

Nutritional Value: Calories: 220 | Phosphorus: 3g | Sodium: 4g | Protein: 4g | Carbohydrates: 25g | Fats: 10g | Potassium: 5g | Iron: 4g

---

Quinoa Tabbouleh with Mint

Prep Time: 15 minutes | **Cook Time**: 15 minutes | **Total Time**: 30 minutes | **Per Serving**: 4 servings

Ingredients:

- 1 cup quinoa, rinsed

- 2 cups water

- 1 cup cherry tomatoes, quartered

- 1 cucumber, diced

- 1/4 red onion, finely chopped

- 1/4 cup fresh parsley, chopped

- 1/4 cup fresh mint, chopped

- 3 tablespoons lemon juice

- 3 tablespoons extra virgin olive oil

- Salt and pepper, to taste

Instructions:

1. In a medium saucepan, bring water to a boil. Add quinoa, reduce heat to low, cover, and simmer for 15 minutes. Fluff with a fork and let cool.

2. In a large bowl, combine cooled quinoa, cherry tomatoes, cucumber, red onion, parsley, and mint.

3. In a small bowl, whisk together lemon juice, olive oil, salt, and pepper.

4. Pour the dressing over the quinoa mixture and toss until well combined.

5. Serve chilled.

Nutritional Value: Calories: 240 | Phosphorus: 4g | Sodium: 5g | Protein: 6g | Carbohydrates: 30g | Fats: 10g | Potassium: 4g | Iron: 5g

---

Lentil and Kale Power Bowl

Prep Time: 10 minutes | **Cook Time**: 30 minutes | **Total Time**: 40 minutes | **Per Serving**: 4 servings

Ingredients:

- 1 cup lentils, rinsed

- 4 cups vegetable broth

- 2 cups kale, chopped

- 1 cup cherry tomatoes, halved

- 1/2 red onion, thinly sliced

- 1 avocado, diced

- 2 tablespoons extra virgin olive oil

- 2 tablespoons lemon juice

- 1 clove garlic, minced

- Salt and pepper, to taste

Instructions:

1. In a large saucepan, combine lentils and vegetable broth. Bring to a boil, reduce heat, and simmer for 20-25 minutes until lentils are tender. Drain any excess liquid.

2. In a large bowl, combine cooked lentils, kale, cherry tomatoes, red onion, and avocado.

3. In a small bowl, whisk together olive oil, lemon juice, garlic, salt, and pepper.

4. Pour the dressing over the lentil mixture and toss until well combined.

5. Serve immediately.

Nutritional Value: Calories: 320 | Phosphorus: 5g | Sodium: 6g | Protein: 12g | Carbohydrates: 35g | Fats: 15g | Potassium: 6g | Iron: 7g

Cucumber and Dill Greek Salad

Prep Time: 10 minutes | **Cook Time**: 0 minutes | **Total Time**: 10 minutes | **Per Serving**: 4 servings

Ingredients:

- 2 cucumbers, diced
- 1/2 red onion, thinly sliced
- 1/4 cup fresh dill, chopped
- 1/4 cup Kalamata olives, pitted
- 1/4 cup feta cheese, crumbled
- 3 tablespoons olive oil
- 2 tablespoons red wine vinegar
- Salt and pepper, to taste

Instructions:

1. In a large bowl, combine cucumbers, red onion, dill, olives, and feta cheese.
2. In a small bowl, whisk together olive oil, red wine vinegar, salt, and pepper.
3. Pour the dressing over the cucumber mixture and toss until well combined.
4. Serve immediately.

Nutritional Value: Calories: 150 | Phosphorus: 3g | Sodium: 5g | Protein: 4g | Carbohydrates: 10g | Fats: 12g | Potassium: 3g | Iron: 2g

Tempeh Reuben Sandwich

Prep Time: 15 minutes | **Cook Time**: 10 minutes | **Total Time**: 25 minutes | **Per Serving**: 4 servings

Ingredients:

- 1 block (8 ounces) tempeh, sliced
- 8 slices rye bread
- 1 cup sauerkraut
- 4 slices Swiss cheese (optional)
- 1/4 cup Thousand Island dressing
- 2 tablespoons olive oil
- 1 tablespoon soy sauce
- 1 tablespoon apple cider vinegar
- 1 teaspoon smoked paprika

Instructions:

1. In a bowl, mix olive oil, soy sauce, apple cider vinegar, and smoked paprika. Marinate tempeh slices in the mixture for 10 minutes.

2. Heat a skillet over medium heat and cook tempeh slices for 3-4 minutes on each side until browned.

3. To assemble the sandwiches, spread Thousand Island dressing on each slice of bread.

4. Layer with tempeh, sauerkraut, and Swiss cheese if using.

5. Close the sandwiches and cook on a skillet or griddle for 2-3 minutes on each side until the bread is toasted and the cheese is melted.

6. Serve immediately.

Nutritional Value: Calories: 350 | Phosphorus: 5g | Sodium: 8g | Protein: 15g | Carbohydrates: 35g | Fats: 18g | Potassium: 4g | Iron: 4g

Edamame and Carrot Ginger Salad

Prep Time: 10 minutes | **Cook Time**: 5 minutes | **Total Time**: 15 minutes | **Per Serving**: 4 servings

Ingredients:

- 1 cup shelled edamame, cooked
- 2 carrots, shredded
- 1/2 red bell pepper, diced
- 1/4 cup fresh cilantro, chopped
- 2 tablespoons sesame seeds
- 2 tablespoons rice vinegar
- 1 tablespoon soy sauce
- 1 tablespoon sesame oil
- 1 teaspoon fresh ginger, grated
- 1 clove garlic, minced
- Salt and pepper, to taste

Instructions:

1. In a large bowl, combine cooked edamame, shredded carrots, red bell pepper, cilantro, and sesame seeds.

2. In a small bowl, whisk together rice vinegar, soy sauce, sesame oil, ginger, garlic, salt, and pepper.

3. Pour the dressing over the salad and toss until well combined.

4. Serve chilled.

Nutritional Value: Calories: 180 | Phosphorus: 3g | Sodium: 6g | Protein: 7g | Carbohydrates: 15g | Fats: 10g | Potassium: 3g | Iron: 3g

Stuffed Bell Peppers with Rice and Beans

Prep Time: 15 minutes | **Cook Time**: 45 minutes | **Total Time**: 60 minutes | **Per Serving**: 4 servings

Ingredients:

- 4 bell peppers, tops cut off and seeds removed
- 1 cup cooked rice
- 1 can (15 ounces) black beans, drained and rinsed
- 1 cup corn kernels
- 1/2 cup salsa
- 1/2 cup shredded cheese (optional)
- 1 teaspoon cumin
- 1/2 teaspoon chili powder
- Salt and pepper, to taste
- 1 tablespoon olive oil

Instructions:

1. Preheat the oven to 375°F (190°C).
2. In a large bowl, mix cooked rice, black beans, corn, salsa, cumin, chili powder, salt, and pepper.
3. Stuff each bell pepper with the rice and bean mixture.
4. Place stuffed peppers in a baking dish and drizzle with olive oil.
5. Cover with foil and bake for 30 minutes.
6. Remove foil, sprinkle with cheese if using, and bake for an additional 15 minutes until peppers are tender.
7. Serve immediately.

Nutritional Value: Calories: 280 | Phosphorus: 4g | Sodium: 5g | Protein: 10g | Carbohydrates: 40g | Fats: 8g | Potassium: 4g | Iron: 5g

Watermelon, Feta, and Arugula Salad

Prep Time: 10 minutes | **Cook Time**: 0 minutes | **Total Time**: 10 minutes | **Per Serving**: 4 servings

Ingredients:

- 4 cups arugula
- 2 cups watermelon, cubed
- 1/2 cup feta cheese, crumbled
- 1/4 red onion, thinly sliced
- 2 tablespoons balsamic glaze
- 2 tablespoons extra virgin olive oil
- Salt and pepper, to taste

Instructions:

1. In a large bowl, combine arugula, watermelon, feta cheese, and red onion.
2. Drizzle with balsamic glaze and olive oil.
3. Season with salt and pepper.
4. Toss gently and serve immediately.

Nutritional Value: Calories: 150 | Phosphorus: 3g | Sodium: 6g | Protein: 4g | Carbohydrates: 15g | Fats: 10g | Potassium: 3g | Iron: 2g

Soups and Stews

Vegetable Minestrone Soup

Prep Time: 15 minutes | **Cook Time**: 30 minutes | **Total Time**: 45 minutes | **Per Serving**: 6 servings

Ingredients:

- 1 tablespoon olive oil
- 1 onion, diced
- 2 cloves garlic, minced
- 2 carrots, diced
- 2 celery stalks, diced
- 1 zucchini, diced
- 1 yellow bell pepper, diced
- 1 can (15 ounces) diced tomatoes
- 4 cups vegetable broth
- 1 can (15 ounces) kidney beans, drained and rinsed
- 1 cup green beans, chopped
- 1/2 cup small pasta (optional)
- 1 teaspoon dried basil
- 1 teaspoon dried oregano
- Salt and pepper, to taste
- 1/4 cup fresh parsley, chopped

Instructions:

1. Heat olive oil in a large pot over medium heat. Add onion and garlic, and sauté until softened.

2. Add carrots, celery, zucchini, and bell pepper. Cook for 5-7 minutes until vegetables begin to soften.

3. Stir in diced tomatoes, vegetable broth, kidney beans, green beans, pasta (if using), basil, and oregano. Bring to a boil.

4. Reduce heat and simmer for 20-25 minutes until vegetables and pasta are tender.

5. Season with salt and pepper to taste.

6. Garnish with fresh parsley and serve hot.

Nutritional Value: Calories: 180 | Phosphorus: 4g | Sodium: 6g | Protein: 6g | Carbohydrates: 28g | Fats: 5g | Potassium: 5g | Iron: 4g

Butternut Squash and Apple Bisque

Prep Time: 15 minutes | **Cook Time**: 30 minutes | **Total Time**: 45 minutes | **Per Serving**: 6 servings

Ingredients:

- 1 tablespoon olive oil
- 1 onion, diced
- 2 cloves garlic, minced
- 1 butternut squash, peeled and cubed
- 2 apples, peeled and chopped
- 4 cups vegetable broth
- 1/2 teaspoon ground cinnamon
- 1/4 teaspoon ground nutmeg
- Salt and pepper, to taste
- 1/2 cup coconut milk

Instructions:

1. Heat olive oil in a large pot over medium heat. Add onion and garlic, and sauté until softened.

2. Add butternut squash and apples. Cook for 5 minutes, stirring occasionally.

3. Pour in vegetable broth, cinnamon, and nutmeg. Bring to a boil.

4. Reduce heat and simmer for 25-30 minutes until squash and apples are tender.

5. Using an immersion blender, puree the soup until smooth.

6. Stir in coconut milk and season with salt and pepper.

7. Serve hot.

Nutritional Value: Calories: 160 | Phosphorus: 3g | Sodium: 5g | Protein: 3g | Carbohydrates: 30g | Fats: 5g | Potassium: 4g | Iron: 3g

Lentil and Spinach Curry Soup

Prep Time: 10 minutes | **Cook Time**: 25 minutes | **Total Time**: 35 minutes | **Per Serving**: 4 servings

Ingredients:

- 1 tablespoon olive oil
- 1 onion, diced
- 2 cloves garlic, minced
- 1 tablespoon ginger, minced
- 1 cup red lentils, rinsed
- 4 cups vegetable broth
- 1 can (14 ounces) coconut milk
- 2 cups spinach, chopped
- 1 tablespoon curry powder
- 1 teaspoon ground cumin
- 1/2 teaspoon turmeric
- Salt and pepper, to taste

Instructions:

1. Heat olive oil in a large pot over medium heat. Add onion, garlic, and ginger, and sauté until softened.
2. Stir in lentils, vegetable broth, coconut milk, curry powder, cumin, and turmeric. Bring to a boil.
3. Reduce heat and simmer for 20 minutes until lentils are tender.
4. Stir in spinach and cook for 2-3 minutes until wilted.
5. Season with salt and pepper.
6. Serve hot.

Nutritional Value: Calories: 250 | Phosphorus: 5g | Sodium: 6g | Protein: 12g | Carbohydrates: 30g | Fats: 10g | Potassium: 5g | Iron: 6g

Tom Yum Gong (Thai Hot and Sour Soup)

Prep Time: 10 minutes | **Cook Time**: 20 minutes | **Total Time**: 30 minutes | **Per Serving**: 4 servings

Ingredients:

- 4 cups chicken or vegetable broth
- 1 stalk lemongrass, cut into 2-inch pieces and smashed
- 3 Thai lime leaves, torn
- 2-3 Thai chilies, smashed
- 1-inch piece galangal, sliced
- 1 cup mushrooms, sliced
- 1/2-pound shrimp, peeled and deveined
- 2 tablespoons fish sauce
- 2 tablespoons lime juice
- 1 tablespoon chili paste
- 1/2 cup cherry tomatoes, halved
- Fresh cilantro, for garnish

Instructions:

1. In a large pot, bring broth to a boil. Add lemongrass, lime leaves, chilies, and galangal. Simmer for 5 minutes.

2. Add mushrooms and cook for another 5 minutes.

3. Add shrimp, fish sauce, lime juice, and chili paste. Cook until shrimp are pink and cooked through.

4. Stir in cherry tomatoes and remove from heat.

5. Garnish with fresh cilantro and serve hot.

Nutritional Value: Calories: 180 | Phosphorus: 4g | Sodium: 7g | Protein: 15g | Carbohydrates: 10g | Fats: 6g | Potassium: 4g | Iron: 2g

White Bean and Kale Soup

Prep Time: 10 minutes | **Cook Time**: 20 minutes | **Total Time**: 30 minutes | **Per Serving**: 4 servings

Ingredients:

- 1 tablespoon olive oil
- 1 onion, diced
- 2 cloves garlic, minced
- 1 carrot, diced
- 2 stalks celery, diced
- 4 cups vegetable broth
- 1 can (15 ounces) white beans, drained and rinsed
- 2 cups kale, chopped
- 1 teaspoon dried thyme
- 1/2 teaspoon dried rosemary
- Salt and pepper, to taste

Instructions:

1. Heat olive oil in a large pot over medium heat. Add onion, garlic, carrot, and celery. Sauté until vegetables are softened.

2. Stir in vegetable broth, white beans, kale, thyme, and rosemary. Bring to a boil.

3. Reduce heat and simmer for 15-20 minutes until vegetables are tender.

4. Season with salt and pepper.

5. Serve hot.

Nutritional Value: Calories: 170 | Phosphorus: 4g | Sodium: 6g | Protein: 8g |Carbohydrates: 25g | Fats: 5g | Potassium: 4g | Iron: 3g

Carrot and Ginger Soup

Prep Time: 10 minutes | **Cook Time**: 25 minutes | **Total Time**: 35 minutes | **Per Serving**: 4 servings

Ingredients:

- 1 tablespoon olive oil
- 1 onion, diced
- 2 cloves garlic, minced
- 1 tablespoon ginger, minced
- 6 large carrots, peeled and sliced
- 4 cups vegetable broth
- 1/2 teaspoon ground cumin
- Salt and pepper, to taste
- 1/4 cup coconut milk

Instructions:

1. Heat olive oil in a large pot over medium heat. Add onion, garlic, and ginger, and sauté until softened.
2. Add carrots and cook for 5 minutes.
3. Pour in vegetable broth and cumin. Bring to a boil.
4. Reduce heat and simmer for 20 minutes until carrots are tender.
5. Using an immersion blender, puree the soup until smooth.
6. Stir in coconut milk and season with salt and pepper.
7. Serve hot.

Nutritional Value: Calories: 150 | Phosphorus: 3g | Sodium: 5g | Protein: 2g | Carbohydrates: 22g | Fats: 7g | Potassium: 3g | Iron: 2g

Mushroom Barley Stew

Prep Time: 15 minutes | **Cook Time**: 45 minutes | **Total Time**: 60 minutes | **Per Serving**: 4 servings

Ingredients:

- 2 tablespoons olive oil
- 1 onion, diced
- 2 cloves garlic, minced
- 2 cups mushrooms, sliced
- 1 carrot, diced
- 2 stalks celery, diced
- 1/2 cup pearl barley
- 4 cups vegetable broth
- 1 teaspoon dried thyme
- 1 bay leaf
- Salt and pepper, to taste
- 1/4 cup fresh parsley, chopped

Instructions:

1. Heat olive oil in a large pot over medium heat. Add onion, garlic, mushrooms, carrot, and celery, and sauté until softened.

2. Stir in barley, vegetable broth, thyme, and bay leaf. Bring to a boil.

3. Reduce heat and simmer for 45 minutes until barley is tender.

4. Season with salt and pepper.

5. Remove bay leaf, garnish with fresh parsley, and serve hot.

Nutritional Value: Calories: 250 | Phosphorus: 5g | Sodium: 6g | Protein: 8g | Carbohydrates: 38g | Fats: 8g | Potassium: 5g | Iron: 4g

Miso Soup with Tofu and Seaweed

Prep Time: 10 minutes | **Cook Time**: 10 minutes | **Total Time**: 20 minutes | **Per Serving**: 4 servings

Ingredients:

- 4 cups water
- 1/4 cup miso paste
- 1/2 cup tofu, cubed
- 1/4 cup seaweed (wakame), soaked and drained
- 1 green onion, sliced

Instructions:

1. In a medium pot, bring water to a simmer.
2. Add miso paste and stir until dissolved.
3. Add tofu and seaweed and cook for 2-3 minutes until heated through.
4. Remove from heat and garnish with sliced green onion.
5. Serve hot.

Nutritional Value: Calories: 80 | Phosphorus: 2g | Sodium: 5g | Protein: 6g | Carbohydrates: 8g | Fats: 3g | Potassium: 3g | Iron: 2g

Gazpacho (Cold Tomato Soup)

Prep Time: 15 minutes | **Cook Time**: 0 minutes | **Total Time**: 15 minutes | **Per Serving**: 4 servings

Ingredients:

- 4 large tomatoes, chopped
- 1 cucumber, peeled and chopped
- 1 red bell pepper, chopped
- 1/2 red onion, chopped
- 2 cloves garlic, minced
- 3 cups tomato juice
- 1/4 cup extra virgin olive oil
- 2 tablespoons red wine vinegar
- Salt and pepper, to taste
- 1/4 cup fresh basil, chopped

Instructions:

1. In a blender or food processor, combine tomatoes, cucumber, bell pepper, red onion, and garlic. Blend until smooth.

2. Add tomato juice, olive oil, and red wine vinegar. Blend again until well combined.

3. Season with salt and pepper to taste.

4. Chill in the refrigerator for at least 1 hour before serving.

5. Garnish with fresh basil and serve cold.

Nutritional Value: Calories: 120 | Phosphorus: 3g | Sodium: 6g | Protein: 2g | Carbohydrates: 15g | Fats: 7g | Potassium: 4g | Iron: 3g

Cauliflower and Leek Soup

Prep Time: 10 minutes | **Cook Time**: 30 minutes | **Total Time**: 40 minutes | **Per Serving**: 4 servings

Ingredients:

- 2 tablespoons olive oil
- 2 leeks, white and light green parts only, sliced
- 2 cloves garlic, minced
- 1 head cauliflower, chopped
- 4 cups vegetable broth
- 1/2 teaspoon dried thyme
- Salt and pepper, to taste
- 1/2 cup unsweetened almond milk

Instructions:

1. Heat olive oil in a large pot over medium heat. Add leeks and garlic, and sauté until softened.
2. Add cauliflower, vegetable broth, and thyme. Bring to a boil.
3. Reduce heat and simmer for 20-25 minutes until cauliflower is tender.
4. Using an immersion blender, puree the soup until smooth.
5. Stir in almond milk and season with salt and pepper.
6. Serve hot.

Nutritional Value: Calories: 140 | Phosphorus: 3g | Sodium: 5g | Protein: 3g | Carbohydrates: 15g | Fats: 8g | Potassium: 4g | Iron: 2g

Fish and Seafood

Grilled Salmon with Lemon and Dill

Prep Time: 10 minutes | **Cook Time**: 15 minutes | **Total Time**: 25 minutes | **Per Serving**: 4 servings

Ingredients:

- 4 salmon fillets
- 2 tablespoons olive oil
- 1 lemon, thinly sliced
- 2 tablespoons fresh dill, chopped
- Salt and pepper, to taste

Instructions:

1. Preheat the grill to medium-high heat.
2. Brush the salmon fillets with olive oil and season with salt and pepper.
3. Place lemon slices on top of each fillet.
4. Grill the salmon for 6-8 minutes per side, or until cooked through.
5. Garnish with fresh dill and serve immediately.

Nutritional Value: Calories: 250 | Phosphorus: 4g | Sodium: 6g | Protein: 22g | Carbohydrates: 1g | Fats: 18g | Potassium: 4g | Iron: 1g

Baked Cod with Cherry Tomatoes

Prep Time: 10 minutes | **Cook Time**: 20 minutes | **Total Time**: 30 minutes | **Per Serving**: 4 servings

Ingredients:

- 4 cod fillets
- 1-pint cherry tomatoes, halved
- 2 cloves garlic, minced
- 2 tablespoons olive oil
- 1/4 cup fresh basil, chopped
- Salt and pepper, to taste

Instructions:

1. Preheat the oven to 400°F (200°C).
2. Place the cod fillets in a baking dish and season with salt and pepper.
3. In a bowl, combine cherry tomatoes, garlic, olive oil, and basil.
4. Pour the tomato mixture over the cod fillets.
5. Bake for 15-20 minutes, or until the fish is cooked through.
6. Serve immediately.

Nutritional Value: Calories: 200 | Phosphorus: 3g | Sodium: 5g | Protein: 25g | Carbohydrates: 5g | Fats: 8g | Potassium: 4g | Iron: 1g

Shrimp Scampi with Zucchini Noodles

Prep Time: 10 minutes | **Cook Time**: 10 minutes | **Total Time**: 20 minutes | **Per Serving**: 4 servings

Ingredients:

- 1 pound shrimp, peeled and deveined
- 3 zucchinis, spiralized
- 3 cloves garlic, minced
- 1/4 cup olive oil
- 1/4 cup white wine
- 1/4 cup fresh parsley, chopped
- Juice of 1 lemon
- Salt and pepper, to taste

Instructions:

1. Heat olive oil in a large skillet over medium heat. Add garlic and sauté until fragrant.
2. Add shrimp and cook until pink, about 2-3 minutes per side.
3. Pour in white wine and lemon juice and cook for another 2 minutes.
4. Add zucchini noodles and toss to combine. Cook until zucchini is just tender.
5. Season with salt and pepper, and garnish with fresh parsley.
6. Serve immediately.

Nutritional Value: Calories: 250 | Phosphorus: 4g | Sodium: 5g | Protein: 28g | Carbohydrates: 7g | Fats: 12g | Potassium: 5g | Iron: 3g

Mussels in White Wine Broth

Prep Time: 10 minutes | **Cook Time**: 10 minutes | **Total Time**: 20 minutes | **Per Serving**: 4 servings

Ingredients:

- 2 pounds mussels, cleaned and debearded
- 2 tablespoons olive oil
- 2 shallots, finely chopped
- 4 cloves garlic, minced
- 1 cup white wine
- 1/2 cup vegetable broth
- 1/4 cup fresh parsley, chopped
- Salt and pepper, to taste

Instructions:

1. Heat olive oil in a large pot over medium heat. Add shallots and garlic, and sauté until softened.
2. Pour in white wine and vegetable broth and bring to a boil.
3. Add mussels, cover, and cook for 5-7 minutes, or until mussels have opened.
4. Discard any mussels that do not open.
5. Season with salt and pepper, and garnish with fresh parsley.
6. Serve immediately.

Nutritional Value: Calories: 220 | Phosphorus: 5g | Sodium: 7g | Protein: 18g | Carbohydrates: 8g | Fats: 8g | Potassium: 4g | Iron: 6g

Tuna Steak with Wasabi Mayo

Prep Time: 10 minutes | **Cook Time**: 10 minutes | **Total Time**: 20 minutes | **Per Serving**: 4 servings

Ingredients:

- 4 tuna steaks
- 2 tablespoons olive oil
- Salt and pepper, to taste
- 1/4 cup mayonnaise
- 1 tablespoon wasabi paste
- 1 tablespoon soy sauce
- 1 teaspoon lemon juice

Instructions:

1. Preheat the grill to high heat.
2. Brush tuna steaks with olive oil and season with salt and pepper.
3. Grill tuna steaks for 2-3 minutes per side, or until desired doneness.
4. In a small bowl, mix mayonnaise, wasabi paste, soy sauce, and lemon juice.
5. Serve tuna steaks topped with wasabi mayo.

Nutritional Value: Calories: 300 | Phosphorus: 4g | Sodium: 6g | Protein: 30g | Carbohydrates: 2g | Fats: 20g | Potassium: 4g | Iron: 2g

Broiled Tilapia with Pesto

Prep Time: 10 minutes | **Cook Time**: 10 minutes | **Total Time**: 20 minutes | **Per Serving**: 4 servings

Ingredients:

- 4 tilapia fillets
- 1/2 cup pesto sauce
- 1 tablespoon olive oil
- Salt and pepper, to taste
- Lemon wedges, for serving

Instructions:

1. Preheat the broiler.
2. Place tilapia fillets on a baking sheet and brush with olive oil. Season with salt and pepper.
3. Spread pesto sauce over each fillet.
4. Broil for 8-10 minutes, or until fish is cooked through.
5. Serve with lemon wedges.

Nutritional Value: Calories: 220 | Phosphorus: 3g | Sodium: 5g | Protein: 23g | Carbohydrates: 1g | Fats: 14g | Potassium: 3g | Iron: 1g

Scallops with Orange and Fennel

Prep Time: 10 minutes | **Cook Time**: 10 minutes | **Total Time**: 20 minutes | **Per Serving**: 4 servings

Ingredients:

- 1-pound scallops

- 2 tablespoons olive oil

- 1 fennel bulb, thinly sliced

- 1 orange, segmented

- 1/4 cup fresh parsley, chopped

- Salt and pepper, to taste

Instructions:

1. Heat olive oil in a large skillet over medium-high heat. Season scallops with salt and pepper.

2. Sear scallops for 2-3 minutes per side, until golden brown and cooked through. Remove from skillet and set aside.

3. In the same skillet, add fennel and cook for 3-4 minutes until softened.

4. Add orange segments and cook for 1-2 minutes until heated through.

5. Return scallops to the skillet to warm.

6. Garnish with fresh parsley and serve immediately.

Nutritional Value: Calories: 200 | Phosphorus: 4g | Sodium: 4g | Protein: 18g | Carbohydrates: 7g | Fats: 10g | Potassium: 4g | Iron: 1g

Trout Almondine

Prep Time: 10 minutes | **Cook Time**: 10 minutes | **Total Time**: 20 minutes | **Per Serving**: 4 servings

Ingredients:

- 4 trout fillets
- 1/4 cup all-purpose flour
- 1/4 cup sliced almonds
- 1/4 cup butter
- 2 tablespoons lemon juice
- 1 tablespoon fresh parsley, chopped
- Salt and pepper, to taste

Instructions:

1. Season trout fillets with salt and pepper, then dredge in flour.

2. In a large skillet, melt butter over medium heat. Add almonds and cook until golden brown.

3. Remove almonds and set aside. Add trout to the skillet and cook for 3-4 minutes per side until golden and cooked through.

4. Return almonds to the skillet and add lemon juice. Cook for 1-2 minutes until warmed through.

5. Garnish with fresh parsley and serve immediately.

Nutritional Value: Calories: 300 | Phosphorus: 4g | Sodium: 5g | Protein: 25g | Carbohydrates: 5g | Fats: 20g | Potassium: 4g | Iron: 1g

Shrimp and Avocado Salad

Prep Time: 15 minutes | **Cook Time**: 5 minutes | **Total Time**: 20 minutes | **Per Serving**: 4 servings

Ingredients:

- 1 pound shrimp, peeled and deveined
- 2 tablespoons olive oil
- 1 avocado, diced
- 1 cucumber, diced
- 1/4 red onion, thinly sliced
- 1/4 cup fresh cilantro, chopped
- Juice of 2 limes
- Salt and pepper, to taste

Instructions:

1. Heat olive oil in a skillet over medium heat. Add shrimp and cook for 2-3 minutes per side until pink and cooked through.

2. In a large bowl, combine shrimp, avocado, cucumber, red onion, and cilantro.

3. Drizzle with lime juice and toss gently.

4. Season with salt and pepper and serve immediately.

Nutritional Value: Calories: 250 | Phosphorus: 4g | Sodium: 5g | Protein: 20g | Carbohydrates: 10g | Fats: 15g | Potassium: 4g | Iron: 2g

Grilled Swordfish with Olive Tapenade

Prep Time: 10 minutes | **Cook Time**: 10 minutes | **Total Time**: 20 minutes | **Per Serving**: 4 servings

Ingredients:

- 4 swordfish steaks
- 2 tablespoons olive oil
- Salt and pepper, to taste
- 1/2 cup olive tapenade
- Lemon wedges, for serving

Instructions:

1. Preheat the grill to medium-high heat.
2. Brush swordfish steaks with olive oil and season with salt and pepper.
3. Grill for 4-5 minutes per side, or until cooked through.
4. Top each steak with a spoonful of olive tapenade.
5. Serve with lemon wedges.

Nutritional Value: Calories: 300 | Phosphorus: 4g | Sodium: 6g | Protein: 28g | Carbohydrates: 2g | Fats: 20g | Potassium: 5g | Iron: 2g

Chicken and Poultry

Herb-Roasted Chicken with Root Vegetables

Prep Time: 15 minutes | **Cook Time**: 60 minutes | **Total Time**: 75 minutes | **Per Serving**: 4 servings

Ingredients:

- 1 whole chicken (about 4 pounds), giblets removed
- 4 tablespoons olive oil, divided
- 1 tablespoon fresh rosemary, chopped
- 1 tablespoon fresh thyme, chopped
- 1 tablespoon fresh sage, chopped
- 3 cloves garlic, minced
- Salt and pepper, to taste
- 4 carrots, peeled and cut into chunks
- 4 parsnips, peeled and cut into chunks
- 2 potatoes, cut into chunks
- 1 onion, quartered

Instructions:

1. Preheat the oven to 375°F (190°C).
2. In a small bowl, mix 2 tablespoons of olive oil, rosemary, thyme, sage, garlic, salt, and pepper.

3. Rub the herb mixture all over the chicken, including under the skin.

4. Toss the root vegetables with the remaining olive oil, salt, and pepper, and place them in a roasting pan.

5. Place the chicken on top of the vegetables.

6. Roast for 60 minutes or until the chicken is cooked through and the vegetables are tender.

7. Let the chicken rest for 10 minutes before carving.

8. Serve the chicken with the roasted vegetables.

Nutritional Value: Calories: 450 | Phosphorus: 5g | Sodium: 6g | Protein: 40g | Carbohydrates: 20g | Fats: 25g | Potassium: 5g | Iron: 3g

Turkey Chili with White Beans

Prep Time: 15 minutes | **Cook Time**: 45 minutes | **Total Time**: 60 minutes | **Per Serving**: 4 servings

Ingredients:

- 1 tablespoon olive oil
- 1 pound ground turkey
- 1 onion, diced
- 2 cloves garlic, minced
- 1 red bell pepper, diced
- 1 can (15 ounces) white beans, drained and rinsed
- 1 can (14.5 ounces) diced tomatoes
- 1 cup chicken broth
- 1 tablespoon chili powder
- 1 teaspoon ground cumin
- 1/2 teaspoon paprika
- Salt and pepper, to taste

Instructions:

1. Heat olive oil in a large pot over medium heat. Add ground turkey, onion, and garlic, and cook until the turkey is browned.

2. Add bell pepper and cook for another 5 minutes.

3. Stir in white beans, diced tomatoes, chicken broth, chili powder, cumin, paprika, salt, and pepper.

4. Bring to a boil, then reduce heat and simmer for 30 minutes.

5. Serve hot.

Nutritional Value: Calories: 300 | Phosphorus: 4g | Sodium: 6g | Protein: 28g | Carbohydrates: 25g | Fats: 10g | Potassium: 5g | Iron: 4g

Lemon Garlic Chicken Skewers

Prep Time: 15 minutes | **Cook Time**: 15 minutes | **Total Time**: 30 minutes | **Per Serving**: 4 servings

Ingredients:

- 1-pound boneless, skinless chicken breasts, cut into 1-inch pieces

- 2 tablespoons olive oil

- Juice of 2 lemons

- 3 cloves garlic, minced

- 1 tablespoon fresh parsley, chopped

- 1 teaspoon dried oregano

- Salt and pepper, to taste

Instructions:

1. In a bowl, combine olive oil, lemon juice, garlic, parsley, oregano, salt, and pepper.

2. Add chicken pieces and toss to coat. Marinate for at least 30 minutes.

3. Preheat the grill to medium-high heat.

4. Thread chicken onto skewers.

5. Grill chicken skewers for 10-15 minutes, turning occasionally, until cooked through.

6. Serve immediately.

Nutritional Value: Calories: 220 | Phosphorus: 3g | Sodium: 4g | Protein: 26g | Carbohydrates: 2g | Fats: 12g | Potassium: 3g | Iron: 1g

Chicken and Quinoa Stuffed Peppers

Prep Time: 20 minutes | **Cook Time**: 30 minutes | **Total Time**: 50 minutes | **Per Serving**: 4 servings

Ingredients:

- 4 bell peppers, tops cut off and seeds removed
- 1 cup cooked quinoa
- 1 pound ground chicken
- 1 onion, diced
- 2 cloves garlic, minced
- 1 cup diced tomatoes
- 1 teaspoon dried oregano
- 1 teaspoon ground cumin
- Salt and pepper, to taste
- 1/2 cup shredded cheese (optional)

Instructions:

1. Preheat the oven to 375°F (190°C).

2. In a skillet, cook ground chicken, onion, and garlic over medium heat until the chicken is cooked through.

3. Stir in cooked quinoa, diced tomatoes, oregano, cumin, salt, and pepper. Cook for 5 minutes.

4. Stuff each bell pepper with the chicken and quinoa mixture.

5. Place stuffed peppers in a baking dish and top with shredded cheese if using.

6. Bake for 25-30 minutes until peppers are tender.

7. Serve immediately.

Nutritional Value: Calories: 280 | Phosphorus: 4g | Sodium: 5g | Protein: 24g | Carbohydrates: 25g | Fats: 10g | Potassium: 4g | Iron: 3g

Turkey Meatballs with Marinara

Prep Time: 15 minutes | **Cook Time**: 30 minutes | **Total Time**: 45 minutes | **Per Serving**: 4 servings

Ingredients:

- 1 pound ground turkey
- 1/2 cup breadcrumbs
- 1/4 cup grated Parmesan cheese
- 1 egg
- 2 cloves garlic, minced
- 2 tablespoons fresh parsley, chopped
- Salt and pepper, to taste
- 2 cups marinara sauce

Instructions:

1. Preheat the oven to 375°F (190°C).
2. In a bowl, combine ground turkey, breadcrumbs, Parmesan cheese, egg, garlic, parsley, salt, and pepper. Mix well.
3. Form the mixture into meatballs and place on a baking sheet.
4. Bake for 20 minutes until meatballs are cooked through.
5. In a pot, heat marinara sauce over medium heat.
6. Add cooked meatballs to the marinara sauce and simmer for 10 minutes.
7. Serve hot.

Nutritional Value: Calories: 320 | Phosphorus: 5g | Sodium: 6g | Protein: 28g | Carbohydrates: 20g | Fats: 15g | Potassium: 4g | Iron: 3g

Chicken Stir-Fry with Snow Peas

Prep Time: 10 minutes | **Cook Time**: 15 minutes | **Total Time**: 25 minutes | **Per Serving**: 4 servings

Ingredients:

- 1-pound boneless, skinless chicken breasts, sliced
- 2 tablespoons soy sauce
- 1 tablespoon sesame oil
- 1 tablespoon olive oil
- 2 cloves garlic, minced
- 1 tablespoon ginger, minced
- 2 cups snow peas
- 1 red bell pepper, sliced
- 1 carrot, julienned
- 1/4 cup chicken broth
- 1 tablespoon cornstarch
- 2 tablespoons water

Instructions:

1. In a bowl, combine chicken slices and soy sauce. Marinate for 10 minutes.

2. In a large skillet or wok, heat sesame oil and olive oil over medium-high heat. Add garlic and ginger, and sauté until fragrant.

3. Add chicken and cook until browned and cooked through.

4. Add snow peas, bell pepper, and carrot. Stir-fry for 3-4 minutes.

5. In a small bowl, mix chicken broth, cornstarch, and water. Pour into the skillet and cook until the sauce thickens.

6. Serve immediately.

Nutritional Value: Calories: 250 | Phosphorus: 4g | Sodium: 5g | Protein: 26g | Carbohydrates: 10g | Fats: 12g | Potassium: 4g | Iron: 2g

Grilled Turkey Breast with Cranberry Salsa

Prep Time: 15 minutes | **Cook Time**: 20 minutes | **Total Time**: 35 minutes | **Per Serving**: 4 servings

Ingredients:

- 1 pound turkey breast, boneless and skinless
- 2 tablespoons olive oil
- Salt and pepper, to taste
- 1 cup fresh cranberries, chopped
- 1/4 red onion, finely chopped
- 1/4 cup fresh cilantro, chopped
- 1 jalapeño, seeded and minced
- Juice of 1 lime
- 1 tablespoon honey

Instructions:

1. Preheat the grill to medium-high heat.
2. Brush turkey breast with olive oil and season with salt and pepper.
3. Grill turkey for 6-8 minutes per side, or until cooked through.
4. In a bowl, combine cranberries, red onion, cilantro, jalapeño, lime juice, and honey.
5. Serve grilled turkey breast topped with cranberry salsa.

Nutritional Value: Calories: 300 | Phosphorus: 5g | Sodium: 4g | Protein: 30g | Carbohydrates: 12g | Fats: 15g | Potassium: 5g | Iron: 2g

Chicken Fajita Bowl with Brown Rice

Prep Time: 15 minutes | **Cook Time**: 25 minutes | **Total Time**: 40 minutes | **Per Serving**: 4 servings

Ingredients:

- 1-pound boneless, skinless chicken breasts, sliced
- 2 tablespoons olive oil
- 1 tablespoon fajita seasoning
- 1 red bell pepper, sliced
- 1 green bell pepper, sliced
- 1 onion, sliced
- 2 cups cooked brown rice
- 1/2 cup salsa
- 1/4 cup fresh cilantro, chopped

Instructions:

1. In a bowl, toss chicken slices with olive oil and fajita seasoning.
2. Heat a large skillet over medium-high heat. Add chicken and cook until browned and cooked through.
3. Add bell peppers and onion and cook until vegetables are tender.
4. Divide brown rice into bowls and top with chicken and vegetable mixture.
5. Garnish with salsa and fresh cilantro.
6. Serve immediately.

Nutritional Value: Calories: 350 | Phosphorus: 5g | Sodium: 6g | Protein: 28g | Carbohydrates: 35g | Fats: 12g | Potassium: 5g | Iron: 3g

Poached Chicken with Asparagus

Prep Time: 10 minutes | **Cook Time**: 20 minutes | **Total Time**: 30 minutes | **Per Serving**: 4 servings

Ingredients:

- 4 boneless, skinless chicken breasts
- 4 cups chicken broth
- 1 lemon, sliced
- 2 cloves garlic, smashed
- 1 bunch asparagus, trimmed
- Salt and pepper, to taste
- 1 tablespoon fresh parsley, chopped

Instructions:

1. In a large pot, bring chicken broth, lemon slices, and garlic to a simmer.
2. Add chicken breasts and poach for 15-20 minutes until cooked through.
3. Remove chicken from the broth and set aside.
4. Add asparagus to the broth and cook for 3-4 minutes until tender.
5. Serve poached chicken with asparagus, seasoned with salt and pepper, and garnished with fresh parsley.

Nutritional Value: Calories: 250 | Phosphorus: 4g | Sodium: 5g | Protein: 30g | Carbohydrates: 5g | Fats: 12g | Potassium: 4g | Iron: 2g

Turkey Lettuce Wraps

Prep Time: 15 minutes | **Cook Time**: 15 minutes | **Total Time**: 30 minutes | **Per Serving**: 4 servings

Ingredients:

- 1 pound ground turkey

- 2 tablespoons olive oil

- 1 onion, diced

- 2 cloves garlic, minced

- 1 tablespoon soy sauce

- 1 tablespoon hoisin sauce

- 1 teaspoon grated ginger

- 1 carrot, julienned

- 1/4 cup green onions, chopped

- 1 head butter lettuce, leaves separated

Instructions:

1. Heat olive oil in a skillet over medium heat. Add ground turkey, onion, and garlic, and cook until the turkey is browned.

2. Stir in soy sauce, hoisin sauce, and grated ginger. Cook for another 5 minutes.

3. Add julienned carrot and green onions and cook for 2-3 minutes.

4. Spoon the turkey mixture into lettuce leaves and serve immediately.

Nutritional Value: Calories: 220 | Phosphorus: 4g | Sodium: 6g | Protein: 24g | Carbohydrates: 8g | Fats: 12g | Potassium: 3g | Iron: 2g

Snacks and Sides

Guacamole with Carrot Sticks

Prep Time: 10 minutes | **Cook Time**: 0 minutes | **Total Time**: 10 minutes | **Per Serving**: 4 servings

Ingredients:

- 3 ripe avocados, peeled and pitted

- 1 lime, juiced

- 1 small onion, finely chopped

- 1 clove garlic, minced

- 1 small tomato, diced

- 1/4 cup fresh cilantro, chopped

- Salt and pepper, to taste

- 4 large carrots, peeled and cut into sticks

Instructions:

1. In a medium bowl, mash the avocados with a fork.

2. Stir in lime juice, onion, garlic, tomato, and cilantro.

3. Season with salt and pepper to taste.

4. Serve immediately with carrot sticks.

Nutritional Value: Calories: 180 | Phosphorus: 3g | Sodium: 4g | Protein: 2g | Carbohydrates: 15g | Fats: 14g | Potassium: 5g | Iron: 1g

Roasted Chickpeas with Paprika

Prep Time: 5 minutes | **Cook Time**: 25 minutes | **Total Time**: 30 minutes | **Per Serving**: 4 servings

Ingredients:

- 1 can (15 ounces) chickpeas, drained and rinsed
- 1 tablespoon olive oil
- 1 teaspoon paprika
- 1/2 teaspoon garlic powder
- 1/2 teaspoon salt
- 1/4 teaspoon black pepper

Instructions:

1. Preheat oven to 400°F (200°C).
2. Pat chickpeas dry with a paper towel.
3. In a bowl, toss chickpeas with olive oil, paprika, garlic powder, salt, and black pepper.
4. Spread chickpeas on a baking sheet in a single layer.
5. Roast for 25 minutes, stirring halfway through, until crispy.
6. Serve immediately.

Nutritional Value: Calories: 120 | Phosphorus: 2g | Sodium: 3g | Protein: 5g | Carbohydrates: 18g | Fats: 4g | Potassium: 2g | Iron: 2g

Sweet Potato Wedges with Aioli

Prep Time: 10 minutes | **Cook Time**: 30 minutes | **Total Time**: 40 minutes | **Per Serving**: 4 servings

Ingredients:

- 2 large, sweet potatoes, cut into wedges
- 2 tablespoons olive oil
- 1 teaspoon smoked paprika
- 1/2 teaspoon garlic powder
- Salt and pepper, to taste
- 1/2 cup mayonnaise
- 1 clove garlic, minced
- 1 tablespoon lemon juice

Instructions:

1. Preheat oven to 425°F (220°C).
2. In a bowl, toss sweet potato wedges with olive oil, smoked paprika, garlic powder, salt, and pepper.
3. Spread wedges on a baking sheet in a single layer.
4. Roast for 25-30 minutes, turning once, until crispy and golden.
5. In a small bowl, mix mayonnaise, minced garlic, and lemon juice to make aioli.
6. Serve sweet potato wedges with aioli.

Nutritional Value: Calories: 250 | Phosphorus: 2g | Sodium: 3g | Protein: 2g | Carbohydrates: 30g | Fats: 14g | Potassium: 4g | Iron: 1g

Hummus with Bell Pepper Slices

Prep Time: 10 minutes | **Cook Time**: 0 minutes | **Total Time**: 10 minutes | **Per Serving**: 4 servings

Ingredients:

- 1 can (15 ounces) chickpeas, drained and rinsed
- 1/4 cup tahini
- 1/4 cup lemon juice
- 2 tablespoons olive oil
- 2 cloves garlic, minced
- 1/2 teaspoon cumin
- Salt and pepper, to taste
- 1/4 cup water (as needed)
- 2 bell peppers, sliced

Instructions:

1. In a food processor, combine chickpeas, tahini, lemon juice, olive oil, garlic, and cumin.
2. Blend until smooth, adding water as needed to reach desired consistency.
3. Season with salt and pepper to taste.
4. Serve hummus with bell pepper slices.

Nutritional Value: Calories: 200 | Phosphorus: 4g | Sodium: 4g | Protein: 6g | Carbohydrates: 20g | Fats: 12g | Potassium: 3g | Iron: 2g

Edamame Pods with Sea Salt

Prep Time: 5 minutes | **Cook Time**: 5 minutes | **Total Time**: 10 minutes | **Per Serving**: 4 servings

Ingredients:

- 2 cups edamame pods
- 1 teaspoon sea salt

Instructions:

1. Bring a large pot of water to a boil. Add edamame pods and cook for 5 minutes.
2. Drain and sprinkle with sea salt.
3. Serve immediately.

Nutritional Value: Calories: 120 | Phosphorus: 2g | Sodium: 3g | Protein: 11g | Carbohydrates: 10g | Fats: 5g | Potassium: 2g | Iron: 1g

Cauliflower Rice Pilaf

Prep Time: 10 minutes | **Cook Time**: 10 minutes | **Total Time**: 20 minutes | **Per Serving**: 4 servings

Ingredients:

- 1 head cauliflower, grated or processed into rice-sized pieces
- 2 tablespoons olive oil
- 1 onion, diced
- 2 cloves garlic, minced
- 1/4 cup slivered almonds, toasted
- 1/4 cup raisins
- 1 teaspoon ground cumin
- Salt and pepper, to taste
- 1/4 cup fresh parsley, chopped

Instructions:

1. In a large skillet, heat olive oil over medium heat. Add onion and garlic, and sauté until softened.

2. Add grated cauliflower and cook for 5-7 minutes until tender.

3. Stir in slivered almonds, raisins, cumin, salt, and pepper.

4. Cook for another 2-3 minutes until heated through.

5. Garnish with fresh parsley and serve immediately.

Nutritional Value: Calories: 150 | Phosphorus: 3g | Sodium: 3g | Protein: 4g | Carbohydrates: 15g | Fats: 9g | Potassium: 3g | Iron: 2g

Air-Fried Zucchini Chips

Prep Time: 10 minutes | **Cook Time**: 15 minutes | **Total Time**: 25 minutes | **Per Serving**: 4 servings

Ingredients:

- 2 medium zucchinis, thinly sliced
- 2 tablespoons olive oil
- 1/4 cup grated Parmesan cheese
- 1/2 teaspoon garlic powder
- Salt and pepper, to taste

Instructions:

1. Preheat the air fryer to 400°F (200°C).
2. In a bowl, toss zucchini slices with olive oil, Parmesan cheese, garlic powder, salt, and pepper.
3. Arrange zucchini slices in a single layer in the air fryer basket.
4. Air fry for 10-15 minutes, shaking the basket halfway through, until crispy and golden.
5. Serve immediately.

Nutritional Value: Calories: 100 | Phosphorus: 2g | Sodium: 2g | Protein: 3g | Carbohydrates: 5g | Fats: 7g | Potassium: 2g | Iron: 1g

Greek Yogurt Dip with Cucumber

Prep Time: 10 minutes | **Cook Time**: 0 minutes | **Total Time**: 10 minutes | **Per Serving**: 4 servings

Ingredients:

- 1 cup Greek yogurt
- 1/2 cucumber, finely chopped
- 1 tablespoon fresh dill, chopped
- 1 clove garlic, minced
- 1 tablespoon lemon juice
- Salt and pepper, to taste

Instructions:

1. In a bowl, mix Greek yogurt, cucumber, dill, garlic, and lemon juice.
2. Season with salt and pepper to taste.
3. Serve immediately or chill until ready to serve.

Nutritional Value: Calories: 80 | Phosphorus: 1g | Sodium: 2g | Protein: 5g | Carbohydrates: 4g | Fats: 3g | Potassium: 1g | Iron: 1g

Quinoa Tabbouleh Side

Prep Time: 15 minutes | **Cook Time**: 15 minutes | **Total Time**: 30 minutes | **Per Serving**: 4 servings

Ingredients:

- 1 cup quinoa, rinsed
- 2 cups water
- 1 cup cherry tomatoes, quartered
- 1 cucumber, diced
- 1/4 red onion, finely chopped
- 1/4 cup fresh parsley, chopped
- 1/4 cup fresh mint, chopped
- 3 tablespoons lemon juice
- 3 tablespoons olive oil
- Salt and pepper, to taste

Instructions:

1. In a medium saucepan, bring water to a boil. Add quinoa, reduce heat to low, cover, and simmer for 15 minutes. Fluff with a fork and let cool.

2. In a large bowl, combine cooled quinoa, cherry tomatoes, cucumber, red onion, parsley, and mint.

3. In a small bowl, whisk together lemon juice, olive oil, salt, and pepper.

4. Pour the dressing over the quinoa mixture and toss until well combined.

5. Serve chilled.

Nutritional Value: Calories: 240 | Phosphorus: 4g | Sodium: 5g | Protein: 6g | Carbohydrates: 30g | Fats: 10g | Potassium: 4g | Iron: 5g

Roasted Brussels Sprouts

Prep Time: 10 minutes | **Cook Time**: 25 minutes | **Total Time**: 35 minutes | **Per Serving**: 4 servings

Ingredients:

- 1 pound Brussels sprouts, trimmed and halved

- 2 tablespoons olive oil

- 1/4 teaspoon salt

- 1/4 teaspoon black pepper

- 1 tablespoon balsamic vinegar (optional)

Instructions:

1. Preheat oven to 400°F (200°C).

2. In a bowl, toss Brussels sprouts with olive oil, salt, and pepper.

3. Spread Brussels sprouts on a baking sheet in a single layer.

4. Roast for 20-25 minutes, stirring halfway through, until golden and crispy.

5. Drizzle with balsamic vinegar if desired.

6. Serve immediately.

Nutritional Value: Calories: 110 | Phosphorus: 3g | Sodium: 3g | Protein: 4g | Carbohydrates: 10g | Fats: 7g | Potassium: 3g | Iron: 2g

Desserts

Baked Apples with Cinnamon

Prep Time: 10 minutes | **Cook Time**: 30 minutes | **Total Time**: 40 minutes | **Per Serving**: 4 servings

Ingredients:

- 4 apples, cored
- 1/4 cup brown sugar
- 1 teaspoon ground cinnamon
- 1/4 cup chopped walnuts (optional)
- 1/4 cup raisins (optional)
- 1 tablespoon butter, cut into small pieces

Instructions:

1. Preheat the oven to 375°F (190°C).
2. Place the apples in a baking dish.
3. In a small bowl, mix brown sugar, cinnamon, walnuts, and raisins.
4. Stuff the mixture into the apples and top each with a piece of butter.
5. Bake for 30 minutes, or until apples are tender.
6. Serve warm.

Nutritional Value: Calories: 180 | Phosphorus: 2g | Sodium: 2g | Protein: 2g | Carbohydrates: 36g | Fats: 6g | Potassium: 3g | Iron: 1g

Dark Chocolate Dipped Strawberries

Prep Time: 10 minutes | **Cook Time**: 0 minutes | **Total Time**: 10 minutes | **Per Serving**: 4 servings

Ingredients:

- 1 cup dark chocolate chips
- 1 tablespoon coconut oil
- 1 pint strawberries, washed and dried

Instructions:

1. In a microwave-safe bowl, melt dark chocolate chips and coconut oil in 30-second intervals, stirring until smooth.
2. Dip each strawberry into the melted chocolate, letting excess drip off.
3. Place dipped strawberries on a parchment-lined baking sheet.
4. Refrigerate until chocolate is set, about 15 minutes.
5. Serve chilled.

Nutritional Value: Calories: 140 | Phosphorus: 2g | Sodium: 1g | Protein: 1g | Carbohydrates: 18g | Fats: 8g | Potassium: 2g | Iron: 2g

Chia Seed Pudding with Mango

Prep Time: 10 minutes | **Cook Time**: 0 minutes | **Total Time**: 10 minutes (plus overnight chilling) | **Per Serving**: 4 servings

Ingredients:

- 1/2 cup chia seeds
- 2 cups almond milk
- 1 tablespoon honey
- 1 teaspoon vanilla extract
- 1 ripe mango, peeled and diced

Instructions:

1. In a bowl, whisk together chia seeds, almond milk, honey, and vanilla extract.
2. Cover and refrigerate overnight, or for at least 4 hours.
3. Stir well before serving.
4. Top with diced mango.
5. Serve chilled.

Nutritional Value: Calories: 200 | Phosphorus: 3g | Sodium: 2g | Protein: 5g | Carbohydrates: 30g | Fats: 8g | Potassium: 3g | Iron: 2g

Grilled Peaches with Yogurt

Prep Time: 5 minutes | **Cook Time**: 5 minutes | **Total Time**: 10 minutes | **Per Serving**: 4 servings

Ingredients:

- 4 peaches, halved and pitted
- 2 tablespoons honey
- 1 teaspoon ground cinnamon
- 1 cup Greek yogurt

Instructions:

1. Preheat the grill to medium-high heat.
2. Brush peach halves with honey.
3. Grill peaches for 2-3 minutes per side, until tender and grill marks appear.
4. Sprinkle with cinnamon.
5. Serve grilled peaches with a dollop of Greek yogurt.

Nutritional Value: Calories: 150 | Phosphorus: 2g | Sodium: 3g | Protein: 6g | Carbohydrates: 28g | Fats: 3g | Potassium: 3g | Iron: 1g

Cherry Almond Clafoutis

Prep Time: 15 minutes | **Cook Time**: 30 minutes | **Total Time**: 45 minutes | **Per Serving**: 4 servings

Ingredients:

- 1 cup cherries, pitted
- 3/4 cup almond flour
- 3/4 cup milk
- 3 eggs
- 1/4 cup honey
- 1 teaspoon vanilla extract
- 1/4 teaspoon almond extract
- 1/4 teaspoon salt

Instructions:

1. Preheat the oven to 350°F (175°C).
2. Grease a baking dish and spread cherries evenly in the dish.
3. In a bowl, whisk together almond flour, milk, eggs, honey, vanilla extract, almond extract, and salt.
4. Pour the batter over the cherries.
5. Bake for 30 minutes, or until set and golden.
6. Serve warm.

Nutritional Value: Calories: 210 | Phosphorus: 2g | Sodium: 2g | Protein: 6g | Carbohydrates: 25g | Fats: 10g | Potassium: 2g | Iron: 1g

Pineapple Sorbet

Prep Time: 10 minutes | **Cook Time**: 0 minutes | **Total Time**: 10 minutes (plus freezing time) | **Per Serving**: 4 servings

Ingredients:

- 1 ripe pineapple, peeled and cubed
- 1/4 cup honey
- 1 tablespoon lemon juice

Instructions:

1. In a blender, combine pineapple, honey, and lemon juice.
2. Blend until smooth.
3. Pour the mixture into a shallow dish and freeze for 4 hours, stirring occasionally.
4. Scoop into bowls and serve.

Nutritional Value: Calories: 120 | Phosphorus: 1g | Sodium: 1g | Protein: 1g | Carbohydrates: 30g | Fats: 0g | Potassium: 2g | Iron: 1g

Oat and Berry Crumble

Prep Time: 15 minutes | **Cook Time**: 30 minutes | **Total Time**: 45 minutes | **Per Serving**: 4 servings

Ingredients:

- 2 cups mixed berries (blueberries, strawberries, raspberries)
- 1/2 cup rolled oats
- 1/4 cup almond flour
- 1/4 cup brown sugar
- 1/4 cup butter, melted
- 1/2 teaspoon cinnamon

Instructions:

1. Preheat the oven to 350°F (175°C).
2. Spread mixed berries in a baking dish.
3. In a bowl, combine rolled oats, almond flour, brown sugar, melted butter, and cinnamon.
4. Sprinkle the oat mixture over the berries.
5. Bake for 30 minutes, or until the topping is golden and the berries are bubbly.
6. Serve warm.

Nutritional Value: Calories: 250 | Phosphorus: 2g | Sodium: 3g | Protein: 3g | Carbohydrates: 35g | Fats: 12g | Potassium: 2g | Iron: 1g

Poached Pears in Red Wine

Prep Time: 10 minutes | **Cook Time**: 30 minutes | **Total Time**: 40 minutes | **Per Serving**: 4 servings

Ingredients:

- 4 pears, peeled and cored
- 1 bottle red wine
- 1/2 cup honey
- 1 cinnamon stick
- 1 vanilla bean, split
- 2 strips orange zest

Instructions:

1. In a large pot, combine red wine, honey, cinnamon stick, vanilla bean, and orange zest. Bring to a simmer.
2. Add pears and poach for 20-30 minutes, until tender.
3. Remove pears and continue to simmer the liquid until reduced by half.
4. Serve pears drizzled with the reduced sauce.

Nutritional Value: Calories: 200 | Phosphorus: 1g | Sodium: 1g | Protein: 1g | Carbohydrates: 40g | Fats: 0g | Potassium: 2g | Iron: 1g

Banana "Nice" Cream

Prep Time: 10 minutes | **Cook Time**: 0 minutes | **Total Time**: 10 minutes | **Per Serving**: 4 servings

Ingredients:

- 4 ripe bananas, sliced and frozen
- 1/2 teaspoon vanilla extract
- 1/4 cup almond milk (optional)

Instructions:

1. In a food processor, blend frozen banana slices until smooth and creamy.
2. Add vanilla extract and almond milk if needed for a smoother consistency.
3. Serve immediately or freeze until ready to serve.

Nutritional Value: Calories: 100 | Phosphorus: 1g | Sodium: 1g | Protein: 1g | Carbohydrates: 27g | Fats: 0g | Potassium: 3g | Iron: 1g

Greek Yogurt Panna Cotta

Prep Time: 15 minutes | **Cook Time**: 5 minutes | **Total Time**: 20 minutes (plus chilling time) | **Per Serving**: 4 servings

Ingredients:

- 1 cup Greek yogurt
- 1 cup milk
- 1/4 cup honey
- 1 teaspoon vanilla extract
- 1 packet gelatin
- 2 tablespoons water

Instructions:

1. In a small bowl, sprinkle gelatin over water and let it sit for 5 minutes.
2. In a saucepan, heat milk and honey until warm (do not boil). Remove from heat and stir in gelatin until dissolved.
3. Stir in vanilla extract.
4. Let the mixture cool slightly, then whisk in Greek yogurt until smooth.
5. Pour into serving dishes and refrigerate for at least 4 hours, or until set.
6. Serve chilled.

Nutritional Value: Calories: 150 | Phosphorus: 2g | Sodium: 2g | Protein: 8g | Carbohydrates: 18g | Fats: 4g | Potassium: 2g | Iron: 1g

Beverages

Tart Cherry Juice Spritzer

Prep Time: 5 minutes | **Cook Time**: 0 minutes | **Total Time**: 5 minutes | **Per Serving**: 4 servings

Ingredients:

- 2 cups tart cherry juice

- 2 cups sparkling water

- 1 tablespoon honey (optional)

- Ice cubes

- Fresh mint leaves, for garnish

Instructions:

1. In a pitcher, combine tart cherry juice and sparkling water.

2. Add honey if desired and stir well.

3. Fill glasses with ice cubes and pour the spritzer over the ice.

4. Garnish with fresh mint leaves.

5. Serve immediately.

Nutritional Value: Calories: 50 | Phosphorus: 1g | Sodium: 1g | Protein: 0g | Carbohydrates: 13g | Fats: 0g | Potassium: 1g | Iron: 0g

Green Tea with Lemon

Prep Time: 5 minutes | **Cook Time**: 5 minutes | **Total Time**: 10 minutes | **Per Serving**: 4 servings

Ingredients:

- 4 cups water
- 4 green tea bags
- 1 lemon, sliced
- 1 tablespoon honey (optional)

Instructions:

1. Bring water to a boil in a pot.
2. Remove from heat and add green tea bags. Steep for 3-5 minutes.
3. Remove tea bags and let tea cool slightly.
4. Pour into cups and add lemon slices.
5. Stir in honey if desired.
6. Serve hot or chilled.

Nutritional Value: Calories: 10 | Phosphorus: 0g | Sodium: 0g | Protein: 0g | Carbohydrates: 3g | Fats: 0g | Potassium: 0g | Iron: 0g

Pineapple and Ginger Smoothie

Prep Time: 10 minutes | **Cook Time**: 0 minutes | **Total Time**: 10 minutes | **Per Serving**: 4 servings

Ingredients:

- 2 cups fresh pineapple chunks
- 1 cup coconut water
- 1-inch piece fresh ginger, peeled and grated
- 1 tablespoon honey (optional)
- Ice cubes

Instructions:

1. In a blender, combine pineapple chunks, coconut water, grated ginger, and honey if desired.
2. Blend until smooth.
3. Add ice cubes and blend again until frothy.
4. Pour into glasses and serve immediately.

Nutritional Value: Calories: 70 | Phosphorus: 1g | Sodium: 1g | Protein: 0g | Carbohydrates: 18g | Fats: 0g | Potassium: 1g | Iron: 0g

Cucumber Mint Water

Prep Time: 5 minutes | **Cook Time**: 0 minutes | **Total Time**: 5 minutes | **Per Serving**: 4 servings

Ingredients:

- 1 cucumber, thinly sliced
- 1/4 cup fresh mint leaves
- 4 cups water
- Ice cubes

Instructions:

1. In a pitcher, combine cucumber slices and fresh mint leaves.
2. Fill with water and stir gently.
3. Let it sit in the refrigerator for at least 1 hour to infuse flavors.
4. Serve chilled with ice cubes.

Nutritional Value: Calories: 0 | Phosphorus: 0g | Sodium: 0g | Protein: 0g | Carbohydrates: 1g | Fats: 0g | Potassium: 0g | Iron: 0g

Hibiscus Iced Tea

Prep Time: 10 minutes | **Cook Time**: 10 minutes | **Total Time**: 20 minutes | **Per Serving**: 4 servings

Ingredients:

- 4 cups water

- 1/2 cup dried hibiscus flowers

- 1/4 cup honey (optional)

- Ice cubes

- Lemon slices, for garnish

Instructions:

1. Bring water to a boil in a pot.

2. Remove from heat and add dried hibiscus flowers. Steep for 10 minutes.

3. Strain the tea into a pitcher and stir in honey if desired.

4. Let it cool to room temperature, then refrigerate until chilled.

5. Serve over ice cubes with lemon slices.

Nutritional Value: Calories: 30 | Phosphorus: 0g | Sodium: 0g | Protein: 0g | Carbohydrates: 8g | Fats: 0g | Potassium: 0g | Iron: 0g

Berry and Spinach Smoothie

Prep Time: 5 minutes | **Cook Time**: 0 minutes | **Total Time**: 5 minutes | **Per Serving**: 4 servings

Ingredients:

- 1 cup mixed berries (strawberries, blueberries, raspberries)
- 1 cup fresh spinach
- 1 banana
- 1 cup almond milk
- 1 tablespoon chia seeds
- Ice cubes

Instructions:

1. In a blender, combine mixed berries, spinach, banana, almond milk, and chia seeds.
2. Blend until smooth.
3. Add ice cubes and blend again until frothy.
4. Pour into glasses and serve immediately.

Nutritional Value: Calories: 90 | Phosphorus: 1g | Sodium: 1g | Protein: 2g | Carbohydrates: 22g | Fats: 1g | Potassium: 1g | Iron: 1g

Turmeric Golden Milk

Prep Time: 5 minutes | **Cook Time**: 5 minutes | **Total Time**: 10 minutes | **Per Serving**: 4 servings

Ingredients:

- 2 cups almond milk
- 1 teaspoon ground turmeric
- 1/2 teaspoon ground ginger
- 1/4 teaspoon ground cinnamon
- 1 tablespoon honey (optional)
- 1 teaspoon vanilla extract

Instructions:

1. In a saucepan, combine almond milk, turmeric, ginger, and cinnamon.
2. Heat over medium heat until warm (do not boil).
3. Remove from heat and stir in honey and vanilla extract.
4. Pour into cups and serve immediately.

Nutritional Value: Calories: 60 | Phosphorus: 1g | Sodium: 1g | Protein: 1g | Carbohydrates: 12g | Fats: 1g | Potassium: 1g | Iron: 1g

Coconut Water with Lime

Prep Time: 5 minutes | **Cook Time**: 0 minutes | **Total Time**: 5 minutes | **Per Serving**: 4 servings

Ingredients:

- 4 cups coconut water
- 2 limes, juiced
- Ice cubes
- Lime slices, for garnish

Instructions:

1. In a pitcher, combine coconut water and lime juice.
2. Stir well and pour into glasses over ice cubes.
3. Garnish with lime slices.
4. Serve immediately.

Nutritional Value: Calories: 30 | Phosphorus: 0g | Sodium: 0g | Protein: 0g | Carbohydrates: 8g | Fats: 0g | Potassium: 0g | Iron: 0g

Apple Cider Vinegar Tonic

Prep Time: 5 minutes | **Cook Time**: 0 minutes | **Total Time**: 5 minutes | **Per Serving**: 4 servings

Ingredients:

- 4 cups water

- 1/4 cup apple cider vinegar

- 2 tablespoons honey

- 1 teaspoon ground cinnamon

- Ice cubes

Instructions:

1. In a pitcher, combine water, apple cider vinegar, honey, and ground cinnamon.

2. Stir well until honey is dissolved.

3. Pour into glasses over ice cubes.

4. Serve immediately.

Nutritional Value: Calories: 20 | Phosphorus: 0g | Sodium: 0g | Protein: 0g | Carbohydrates: 5g | Fats: 0g | Potassium: 0g | Iron: 0g

Watermelon and Basil Cooler

Prep Time: 10 minutes | **Cook Time**: 0 minutes | **Total Time**: 10 minutes | **Per Serving**: 4 servings

Ingredients:

- 4 cups watermelon, cubed
- 1/4 cup fresh basil leaves
- 1 tablespoon honey (optional)
- 1 tablespoon lime juice
- Ice cubes

Instructions:

1. In a blender, combine watermelon, basil leaves, honey, and lime juice.
2. Blend until smooth.
3. Pour into glasses over ice cubes.
4. Serve immediately.

Nutritional Value: Calories: 50 | Phosphorus: 1g | Sodium: 1g | Protein: 1g | Carbohydrates: 12g | Fats: 0g | Potassium: 1g | Iron: 1g

Meal Plan

Day 1:

- Breakfast: Almond Butter and Banana Whole Wheat Toast
- Lunch: Mediterranean Chickpea Salad
- Dinner: Herb-Roasted Chicken with Root Vegetables
- Snack: Guacamole with Carrot Sticks

Day 2:

- Breakfast: Greek Yogurt Parfait with Berries and Nuts
- Lunch: Grilled Tofu with Pineapple Salsa
- Dinner: Turkey Chili with White Beans
- Snack: Roasted Chickpeas with Paprika

Day 3:

- Breakfast: Spinach and Mushroom Frittata
- Lunch: Roasted Beet and Orange Salad
- Dinner: Lemon Garlic Chicken Skewers
- Snack: Sweet Potato Wedges with Aioli

Day 4:

- Breakfast: Steel-Cut Oats with Cinnamon and Apples
- Lunch: Quinoa Tabbouleh with Mint
- Dinner: Chicken and Quinoa Stuffed Peppers

- Snack: Hummus with Bell Pepper Slices

Day 5:

- Breakfast: Sweet Potato Hash with Bell Peppers

- Lunch: Lentil and Kale Power Bowl

- Dinner: Turkey Meatballs with Marinara

- Snack: Edamame Pods with Sea Salt

Day 6:

- Breakfast: Cherry Almond Overnight Oats

- Lunch: Cucumber and Dill Greek Salad

- Dinner: Chicken Stir-Fry with Snow Peas

- Snack: Cauliflower Rice Pilaf

Day 7:

- Breakfast: Avocado Toast with Smoked Salmon

- Lunch: Tempeh Reuben Sandwich

- Dinner: Grilled Turkey Breast with Cranberry Salsa

- Snack: Air-Fried Zucchini Chips

Day 8:

- Breakfast: Egg White and Vegetable Wrap

- Lunch: Edamame and Carrot Ginger Salad

- Dinner: Chicken Fajita Bowl with Brown Rice

- Snack: Greek Yogurt Dip with Cucumber

Day 9:

- Breakfast: Quinoa Breakfast Bowl with Mango

- Lunch: Stuffed Bell Peppers with Rice and Beans

- Dinner: Poached Chicken with Asparagus

- Snack: Quinoa Tabbouleh Side

Day 10:

- Breakfast: Zucchini Bread Muffins

- Lunch: Watermelon, Feta, and Arugula Salad

- Dinner: Turkey Lettuce Wraps

- Snack: Roasted Brussels Sprouts

Day 11:

- Breakfast: Almond Butter and Banana Whole Wheat Toast

- Lunch: Vegetable Minestrone Soup

- Dinner: Grilled Salmon with Lemon and Dill

- Snack: Baked Apples with Cinnamon

Day 12:

- Breakfast: Greek Yogurt Parfait with Berries and Nuts

- Lunch: Butternut Squash and Apple Bisque

- Dinner: Baked Cod with Cherry Tomatoes

- Snack: Dark Chocolate Dipped Strawberries

Day 13:

- Breakfast: Spinach and Mushroom Frittata

- Lunch: Lentil and Spinach Curry Soup

- Dinner: Shrimp Scampi with Zucchini Noodles

- Snack: Chia Seed Pudding with Mango

Day 14:

- Breakfast: Steel-Cut Oats with Cinnamon and Apples

- Lunch: Tom Yum Goong (Thai Hot and Sour Soup)

- Dinner: Mussels in White Wine Broth

- Snack: Grilled Peaches with Yogurt

Day 15:

- Breakfast: Sweet Potato Hash with Bell Peppers

- Lunch: White Bean and Kale Soup

- Dinner: Tuna Steak with Wasabi Mayo

- Snack: Cherry Almond Clafoutis

Day 16:

- Breakfast: Cherry Almond Overnight Oats

- Lunch: Carrot and Ginger Soup

- Dinner: Broiled Tilapia with Pesto

- Snack: Pineapple Sorbet

Day 17:

- Breakfast: Avocado Toast with Smoked Salmon

- Lunch: Mushroom Barley Stew

- Dinner: Scallops with Orange and Fennel

- Snack: Oat and Berry Crumble

Day 18:

- Breakfast: Egg White and Vegetable Wrap

- Lunch: Miso Soup with Tofu and Seaweed

- Dinner: Trout Almondine

- Snack: Poached Pears in Red Wine

Day 19:

- Breakfast: Quinoa Breakfast Bowl with Mango

- Lunch: Gazpacho (Cold Tomato Soup)

- Dinner: Shrimp and Avocado Salad

- Snack: Banana "Nice" Cream

Day 20:

- Breakfast: Zucchini Bread Muffins

- Lunch: Cauliflower and Leek Soup

- Dinner: Grilled Swordfish with Olive Tapenade

- Snack: Greek Yogurt Panna Cotta

Day 21:

- Breakfast: Almond Butter and Banana Whole Wheat Toast

- Lunch: Mediterranean Chickpea Salad

- Dinner: Herb-Roasted Chicken with Root Vegetables

- Snack: Tart Cherry Juice Spritzer

Week 4:

Day 22:

- Breakfast: Greek Yogurt Parfait with Berries and Nuts

- Lunch: Grilled Tofu with Pineapple Salsa

- Dinner: Turkey Chili with White Beans

- Snack: Green Tea with Lemon

Day 23:

- Breakfast: Spinach and Mushroom Frittata

- Lunch: Roasted Beet and Orange Salad

- Dinner: Lemon Garlic Chicken Skewers

- Snack: Pineapple and Ginger Smoothie

Day 24:

- Breakfast: Steel-Cut Oats with Cinnamon and Apples

- Lunch: Quinoa Tabbouleh with Mint

- Dinner: Chicken and Quinoa Stuffed Peppers

- Snack: Cucumber Mint Water

Day 25:

- Breakfast: Sweet Potato Hash with Bell Peppers

- Lunch: Lentil and Kale Power Bowl

- Dinner: Turkey Meatballs with Marinara

- Snack: Hibiscus Iced Tea

Day 26:

- Breakfast: Cherry Almond Overnight Oats

- Lunch: Cucumber and Dill Greek Salad

- Dinner: Chicken Stir-Fry with Snow Peas

- Snack: Berry and Spinach Smoothie

Day 27:

- Breakfast: Avocado Toast with Smoked Salmon

- Lunch: Tempeh Reuben Sandwich

- Dinner: Grilled Turkey Breast with Cranberry Salsa

- Snack: Turmeric Golden Milk

Day 28:

- Breakfast: Egg White and Vegetable Wrap

- Lunch: Edamame and Carrot Ginger Salad

- Dinner: Chicken Fajita Bowl with Brown Rice

- Snack: Coconut Water with Lime

Day 29:

- Breakfast: Quinoa Breakfast Bowl with Mango

- Lunch: Stuffed Bell Peppers with Rice and Beans

- Dinner: Poached Chicken with Asparagus

- Snack: Apple Cider Vinegar Tonic

Day 30:

- Breakfast: Zucchini Bread Muffins

- Lunch: Watermelon, Feta, and Arugula Salad

- Dinner: Turkey Lettuce Wraps

- Snack: Watermelon and Basil Cooler

Tips for Dining Out

1. Plan:

- **Research Menus**: Check the restaurant's menu online before you go. Look for options that are low in purines and rich in vegetables and lean proteins.

- **Call Ahead**: If you're unsure about menu options, call the restaurant and ask about how they prepare their dishes or if they can accommodate special dietary needs.

2. Choose the Right Protein:

- **Lean Proteins**: Opt for lean proteins like chicken, turkey, and fish. Avoid high-purine meats such as organ meats, red meats, and shellfish.

- **Vegetarian Options**: Consider vegetarian dishes that use tofu, tempeh, or legumes as protein sources.

3. Focus on Vegetables:

- **Salads and Sides**: Choose salads with a variety of vegetables and a vinaigrette dressing. Avoid creamy dressings that may be high in fats.

- **Roasted and Steamed Vegetables**: Look for dishes that feature roasted, grilled, or steamed vegetables. These are often lower in calories and fats and provide essential nutrients.

4. Be Mindful of Sauces and Additives:

- **Sauces**: Ask for sauces and dressings on the side. Choose options that are broth-based or made with fresh ingredients rather than creamy or rich sauces.

- **Avoid High-Fructose Corn Syrup**: Steer clear of dishes or beverages with high-fructose corn syrup, which can contribute to higher uric acid levels.

5. Watch Portion Sizes:

- **Sharing**: Consider sharing an entrée with a friend or ordering a half-portion if the restaurant offers it.

- **Appetizers as Main Course**: Choose a couple of healthy appetizers as your main meal to control portion size and variety.

6. Drink Wisely:

- **Water**: Drink plenty of water before, during, and after your meal to help flush out uric acid.

- **Avoid Alcohol**: Limit or avoid alcohol, especially beer and liquor, as they can trigger gout flare-ups. If you choose to drink, opt for a small glass of wine instead.

7. Dessert Choices:

- **Fruit-Based Desserts**: Choose desserts that feature fresh fruits rather than rich, sugary options.

- **Small Portions**: If you decide to indulge, consider sharing a dessert or choosing a smaller portion size.

8. Special Requests:

- **Customization**: Don't hesitate to ask for modifications to your meal. Most restaurants are willing to accommodate dietary needs, such as grilling instead of frying or using olive oil instead of butter.

- **Ingredient Substitutions**: Request substitutions, like extra vegetables instead of starchy sides or a whole grain option if available.

Lifestyle Tips

Regular exercise is essential for maintaining health and well-being, especially for seniors. Engaging in physical activity offers numerous benefits, including managing chronic conditions like gout, enhancing mobility, and improving mental health. Here are some key reasons why regular exercise is important for seniors:

1. Improved Joint Health:

- **Reduced Inflammation**: Regular exercise helps reduce inflammation in the joints, which is beneficial for managing conditions like gout.

- **Increased Flexibility**: Stretching and low-impact exercises improve flexibility and range of motion, reducing stiffness and discomfort in the joints.

2. Weight Management:

- **Healthy Weight**: Maintaining a healthy weight is crucial for managing gout, as excess weight can increase uric acid levels and pressure on the joints.

- **Calorie Burn**: Physical activity helps burn calories and prevents weight gain, promoting overall health and reducing the risk of gout flare-ups.

3. Enhanced Cardiovascular Health:

- **Heart Health**: Regular exercise strengthens the heart and improves circulation, reducing the risk of heart disease, hypertension, and stroke.

- **Blood Pressure**: Physical activity helps lower blood pressure, which is essential for overall cardiovascular health.

4. Muscle Strength and Endurance:

- **Muscle Maintenance**: Strength training exercises help maintain muscle mass, which is vital for balance and preventing falls.

- **Increased Endurance**: Regular exercise improves endurance, allowing seniors to perform daily activities with greater ease and less fatigue.

5. Bone Health:

- **Bone Density**: Weight-bearing exercises such as walking and resistance training help maintain bone density and reduce the risk of osteoporosis.

- **Fracture Prevention**: Strong bones are less prone to fractures, which is particularly important for seniors who are at a higher risk of falls.

6. Mental Health Benefits:

- **Reduced Stress**: Exercise is a natural stress reliever, reducing levels of stress hormones and promoting relaxation.

- **Improved Mood**: Physical activity stimulates the production of endorphins, which improve mood and reduce feelings of depression and anxiety.

- **Cognitive Function**: Regular exercise has been shown to improve cognitive function and reduce the risk of cognitive decline and dementia.

7. Enhanced Mobility and Balance:

- **Better Balance**: Exercises that focus on balance and coordination, such as yoga and tai chi, help prevent falls and improve stability.

- **Mobility**: Regular physical activity keeps the body flexible and mobile, making it easier to perform everyday tasks.

8. Social Engagement:

- **Group Activities**: Participating in group exercise classes or sports can provide social interaction, reducing feelings of loneliness and isolation.

- **Community Involvement**: Engaging in community fitness programs helps seniors stay connected and engaged with others.

9. Chronic Disease Management:

- **Blood Sugar Control**: Exercise helps regulate blood sugar levels, which is important for managing diabetes.

- **Reduced Risk**: Regular physical activity reduces the risk of developing chronic diseases such as heart disease, stroke, and certain cancers.

10. Longevity:

- **Increased Lifespan**: Seniors who engage in regular exercise tend to live longer, healthier lives with a better quality of life.

Tips for Incorporating Exercise into Daily Routine:

1. **Start Slowly**: Begin with low-impact exercises and gradually increase the intensity and duration as fitness improves.

2. **Choose Enjoyable Activities**: Select activities that are enjoyable to ensure consistency, such as walking, swimming, gardening, or dancing.

3. **Stay Consistent**: Aim for at least 30 minutes of moderate exercise most days of the week.

4. **Mix It Up**: Include a variety of exercises to work different muscle groups and prevent boredom. Combine aerobic activities, strength training, and flexibility exercises.

5. **Stay Hydrated**: Drink plenty of water before, during, and after exercise to stay hydrated.

6. **Listen to Your Body**: Pay attention to how the body feels during exercise. If there is pain or discomfort, stop and rest.

Managing stress is crucial for overall health and well-being, especially for seniors. Chronic stress can exacerbate health issues, including gout, heart disease, and mental health conditions. Here are effective stress management techniques that seniors can incorporate into their daily lives:

1. Practice Mindfulness and Meditation:

- **Mindfulness**: Engage in mindfulness practices that focus on the present moment. This can help reduce anxiety and improve mental clarity.

- **Meditation**: Daily meditation, even for just a few minutes, can lower stress levels and promote relaxation. Guided meditation apps or videos can be helpful.

2. Deep Breathing Exercises:

- **Breathing Techniques**: Practice deep breathing exercises, such as diaphragmatic breathing or the 4-7-8 technique, to calm the nervous system.

- **Relaxation Response**: Deep breathing can trigger the body's relaxation response, reducing stress hormones and promoting a sense of calm.

3. Social Connections:

- **Stay Connected**: Maintain social connections with family, friends, and community groups. Social interactions provide emotional support and a sense of belonging.

- **Join Groups**: Participate in group activities or clubs that align with your interests, such as book clubs, gardening groups, or senior centers.

4. Hobbies and Interests:

- **Engage in Hobbies**: Spend time on hobbies and activities that bring joy and fulfillment, such as painting, knitting, gardening, or playing musical instruments.

- **Learn Something New**: Take up new hobbies or learn new skills to keep the mind engaged and distracted from stress.

5. Maintain a Healthy Diet:

- **Balanced Nutrition**: Eat a balanced diet rich in fruits, vegetables, whole grains, lean proteins, and healthy fats. Proper nutrition can positively affect mood and energy levels.

- **Hydration**: Stay hydrated by drinking plenty of water throughout the day.

6. Adequate Sleep:

- **Sleep Routine**: Establish a regular sleep routine by going to bed and waking up at the same time each day.

- **Sleep Environment**: Create a comfortable sleep environment that is cool, dark, and quiet. Avoid screens and stimulating activities before bedtime.

7. Limit Stimulants:

- **Reduce Caffeine**: Limit the intake of caffeine and alcohol, as they can increase anxiety and disrupt sleep patterns.

- **Avoid Nicotine**: Refrain from smoking or using tobacco products, which can elevate stress levels.

8. Time Management:

- **Prioritize Tasks**: Break tasks into smaller, manageable steps and prioritize them. Focus on completing one task at a time to avoid feeling overwhelmed.

- **Set Boundaries**: Learn to say no to activities or requests that cause excessive stress or exceed your capacity.

9. Seek Professional Help:

- **Therapy**: Consider talking to a therapist or counselor who can provide strategies and support for managing stress.

- **Support Groups**: Join support groups for individuals facing similar life challenges or health conditions.

10. Relaxation Techniques:

- **Progressive Muscle Relaxation**: Practice progressive muscle relaxation by tensing and then relaxing each muscle group in the body.

- **Guided Imagery**: Use guided imagery or visualization techniques to imagine a peaceful scene or situation, promoting relaxation and stress relief.

11. Engage with Nature:

- **Nature Walks**: Spend time outdoors in nature, whether it's walking in a park, gardening, or simply sitting outside. Nature has a calming effect and can reduce stress.

- **Green Spaces**: Visit green spaces and natural environments regularly to enjoy the benefits of fresh air and natural surroundings.

12. Journaling:

- **Expressive Writing**: Write about your thoughts and feelings in a journal. This can help process emotions and reduce stress.

- **Gratitude Journal**: Keep a gratitude journal to focus on positive aspects of life and cultivate a positive mindset.

13. Laughter and Humor:

- **Laughter**: Engage in activities that make you laugh, such as watching a comedy, reading humorous books, or spending time with funny friends.

- **Humor**: Incorporate humor into your daily life to lighten your mood and reduce stress.